The
Brains
of
Animals
and
Man

Also by the Same Authors

HOW ANIMALS LEARN

ANIMAL INSTINCTS

The
Brains
of
Animals
and
Man

Russell Freedman &
James E. Morriss

Holiday House, Inc. / New York

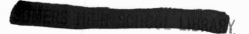

Drawings by James Caraway
Design by Millicent Fairhurst

Copyright © 1972 by Russell Freedman and James E. Morriss
All rights reserved
Printed in the United States of America
Library of Congress catalog card number: 71-154754
ISBN 0-8234-0205-3

to

GEORGE WELLER

who listened . . . and listened . . . and listened

Contents

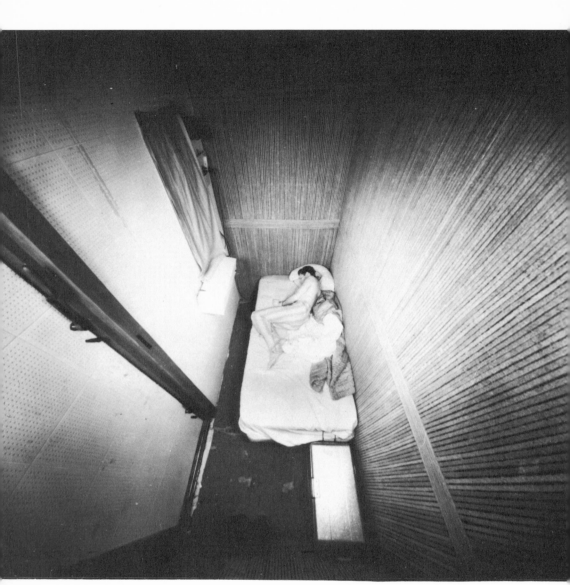

Inside the black room: unaware that he is being photographed by the light of infrared rays, Princeton student Tom Wonnacott lies on the bed in a soundproofed, pitch-black isolation cell. Heavy mittens blunt his sense of touch. At the foot of the bed is a refrigerator containing food.

CHAPTER *1*

The Living Brain

In a dark, cell-like room, a young man lies silently on a bed, arms folded across his chest. He is trying to think, but he finds it difficult to concentrate. Instead, his mind keeps wandering.

Suddenly, in a corner of the room, he notices something move. Sitting up, he leans forward, peers into the corner, and sees a pair of small eyes gleaming. It is an animal . . . a giant squirrel . . . no, a parade of giant squirrels. They have sacks slung over their shoulders and they are marching directly toward him.

Startled, he shakes his head. The squirrels vanish. Then he leans back against the wall and stares into the surrounding darkness.

The room is pitch black. He can see nothing—not even his hand moved back and forth before his eyes. Except for his own breathing, he can hear nothing. He wonders what time it is, what *day* it is. No matter how hard he tries, he cannot remember how long he has been here.

Along with other student volunteers, the young man is taking part in an experiment. Each student has agreed to spend several days in dark, silent isolation. What happens when a person is cut off from the sights, sounds, and sensations of the world around him? How does his mind react?

The Mind in Isolation

Isolation experiments have been conducted at Princeton University in New Jersey, at McGill University in Montreal, Canada, and at other research centers. Although the experimental setup differed from one laboratory to the next, the results were very much the same. Scientists found that a mind in isolation can no longer function normally.

The Princeton experiments were conducted by Dr. Jack Vernon and his co-workers. Here, dozens of student volunteers spent up to four days in a special isolation chamber—a lightproof, soundproof cell called "the black room" where there was nothing to see and nothing to hear. Each volunteer wore heavy mittens which blunted his sense of touch. His only contact with the outside world came during those brief moments when food was brought to the isolation cell.

Most of the volunteers at both Princeton and McGill intended at first to make good use of their time. With nothing to do but lie on their beds and think, they expected to plan term papers in their heads or to make mental notes on courses they were taking. When the experiments got underway, however, they found it impossible to think clearly. In the silent darkness, their minds seemed to drift.

Some volunteers had been told to concentrate on something definite whenever this happened. One student, for instance, was asked to picture a pen in his mind. After a while, he found that this was not easy to do. When he tried to visualize a pen, he saw instead in his mind an ink blot on a white tablecloth. Then he saw a pencil. Then a green horse. Only after great effort was he able to bring a pen to mind.

Before long, many volunteers began to experience "blank periods," when they couldn't focus their thoughts on anything. But the blank periods didn't last. The mind does not stay idle long, for a brain deprived of information soon begins to supply its own. One student was surprised to find: "My mind became full of sounds and colors, and I could not control it." Others heard people talking, or music playing, or choirs singing—and all in stereophonic sound.

Vivid images also appeared to many of the volunteers. It was almost like having dreams while being wide awake. Some of these hallucinations resembled animated movie cartoons: rows of little orange men wearing black caps; prehistoric animals roaming through the jungle; eyeglasses marching down the street; giant squirrels parading with sacks over their shoulders. One student saw pictures of babies flashed on an imaginary screen. Another saw beautiful landscapes. And a third saw a shining doorknob. When he reached out to touch it, he felt a terrific electric shock.

The volunteers seemed to have little control over these hallucinations. Though they might try to rid their minds of them, the same mental images kept turning up over and over again. In fact, some volunteers complained that their eyes became tired from looking at the imaginary pictures.

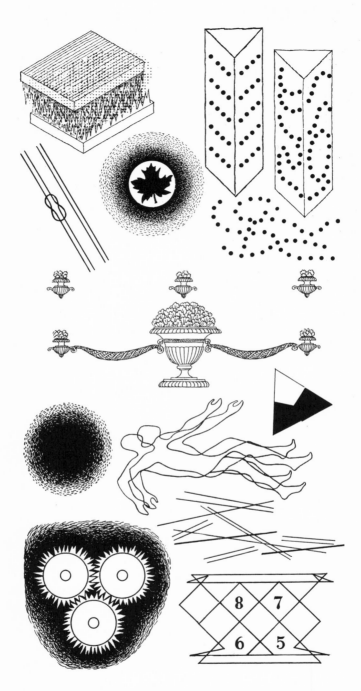

Hallucinations occur frequently among volunteers taking part in sensory deprivation experiments. These drawings depict some of the "images" seen by students who spent long periods in a special isolation cell at McGill University. *From "The Pathology of Boredom," Woodburn Heron. Copyright © 1957 by Scientific American, Inc. All rights reserved.*

Similar hallucinations are sometimes experienced by people who must endure lengthy periods of monotony. Long-distance truck drivers may see imaginary animals running across the road or giant spiders on their windshields. Pilots have also reported hallucinations during long, boring flights. It is possible that prolonged monotony may be responsible for some unexplained plane, train, and automobile accidents.

As the experiments continued, many volunteers experienced weird feelings of "otherness" or "body strangeness." Some reported the sensation of having two bodies. Others felt that their bodies had merged with their beds, or that their minds were floating in space. "My mind seemed to be a ball of cotton floating above my body," said one student. Another reported, "Something seemed to be sucking my mind out through my eyes."

The volunteers also became emotionally unsettled. They grew more and more irritable as time went on and were likely to lose their tempers for no apparent reason. Yet they also had giggling fits and spells of uncontrollable giddiness. They expressed surprise that their feelings could change so much. They seemed to lose all sense of perspective.

When the time finally came for the volunteers to leave their isolation cells, they found it difficult to tune back into the real world. Everything looked distorted. Flat surfaces appeared curved. Objects seemed to change their size and shape. At times, the whole room seemed to be in motion.

The volunteers' ability to peform simple tasks had also been affected by their isolation. Before the Princeton

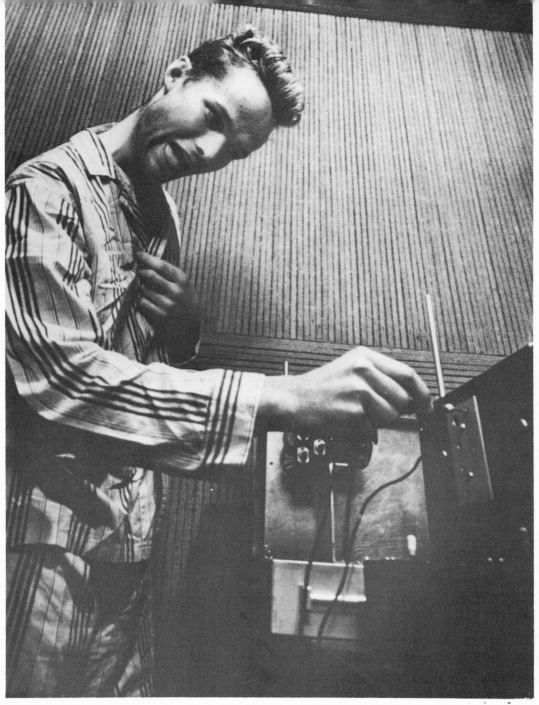

After enduring four days of isolation, student volunteer Wonnacott tries to push a rod through a hole without touching the sides. Despite his agonizing efforts, he failed to perform this simple task.

experiments began, each volunteer had been asked to push a small plastic rod through a hole without touching the sides of the hole. The students considered this an absurdly simple task and succeeded with no effort·at all. After several days in isolation, with their minds deprived of normal stimulation, they were asked to push the same rod through the same hole. This time the task required great effort, and even then many students failed. It was several days before the volunteers returned to normal.

From these experiments, scientists have learned that a steady flow of information coming in through the senses is needed to keep the mind on an even keel. Ordinarily, our brains are constantly stimulated by signals pouring in from the world around us. Without the sights, sounds, and sensations that make up our daily experiences, the mind cannot function normally.

Birthright of the Living Brain

Human beings actively seek stimulation from the world around them. During the experiments at Princeton and McGill, volunteers often talked or sang to themselves in a desperate attempt to gain relief from their long hours of monotonous isolation. They tried to remember in precise detail motion pictures they had seen; they made up imaginary journeys to familiar places; they counted numbers steadily into the thousands. Prisoners kept in solitary confinement often behave in exactly the same way.

Children suffering from blindness, deafness, and other defects of the senses will often attempt to stimulate themselves in strange ways. A blind child may look directly at the sun and move his fingers back and forth before his eyes. He may continue to do this for hours. Apparently, he receives some faint visual sensation, similar perhaps to the sensation you would receive if you closed your eyes and did the same thing. Deaf children sometimes slap their ears or bang their heads as if to force vibrations from their silent worlds.

Like humans, animals also actively seek stimulation. In a famous experiment conducted by psychologist Robert A. Butler, a monkey was placed in a special isolation box. The box was like a small dark cell that contained nothing to interest its inhabitant. One wall of the box had a tiny window through which the monkey could view the world outside. In order to look out, however, he had to open a small door that covered the window. Since the door closed automatically, the monkey had to reopen it every time he wanted to see what was going on outside.

A room with a view: placed in a dark box, this monkey quickly learned to open the window so he could watch what was going on outside. Animals and humans alike actively seek stimulation from their surroundings.

Allan C. Bradbury

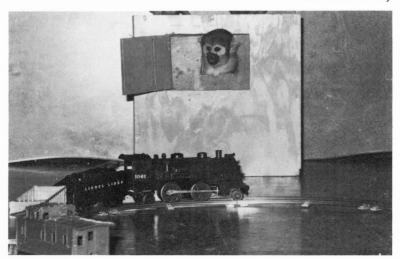

The monkey didn't spend much time in the monotonous darkness of his cell. He quickly learned to open the window and he kept opening it time after time. He would look out frequently to see motionless objects, such as a bowl of fruit. But he would look out even more often to watch moving objects that provided more stimulation, such as a toy train running around a track.

Monkeys, of course, are known for their curiosity. However, other animals will also attempt to avoid monotonous situations. A laboratory rat who has learned to run through a maze in order to find food will take different routes to the food goal if they are available rather than use the same route all the time. The rat will avoid areas where he has spent a good deal of time in order to explore less familiar areas.

Young animals and humans are especially active and curious. Since so many living creatures seek stimulation through their senses from an early age, scientists began to suspect that the brain needs such stimulation in order to develop normally. At the University of California in Berkeley, psychologists Edward L. Bennett and Mark Rosenzweig experimented with two groups of baby gerbils. As soon as the young animals were weaned from their mothers, one group was placed in a large cage where they had plenty of room to run about and lots of toys to play with. They had tunnels to explore, levers to press, ladders to climb, wheels to turn, and a variety of other interesting objects to touch, smell, and see. These gerbils were tamed by their attendants and were frequently picked up and handled.

Unlike their brothers and sisters who grew up in an

enriched and exciting environment, the second group of gerbils grew up alone in small, empty, dimly lit cages. They had no playmates and no room in their cramped quarters to scamper about and explore. They were not handled by their attendants and their barren cages provided them with little or no stimulation.

When all the gerbils were fully grown, they were tested. Those raised in an enriched environment turned out to be much smarter than their deprived brothers and sisters. They were able to learn faster and remember longer than gerbils raised under monotonous, uneventful conditions.

At the end of the experiment, the animals' brains were chemically analyzed, measured, and compared. Scientists found that the privileged gerbils actually had thicker and heavier brains. Although both groups of gerbils had the same number of nerve cells in their brains, the cells were larger and more complex in the brains of gerbils who had grown up in a stimulating environment. These brain cells received a richer supply of blood and contained greater amounts of chemical enzymes that are essential for the brain's normal functioning. By controlling the kind of world the animals grew up in, it was possible to create gerbils with stunted brains and gerbils with healthy, robust, active brains.

Recent studies indicate that stimulation through the senses is just as important to the development of the human brain. In Washington, D.C., a project conducted by the National Institute of Mental Health showed that the IQ's of underprivileged infants can be raised dramatically. When the project began, all the infants were fifteen months old. They were divided into two groups. One

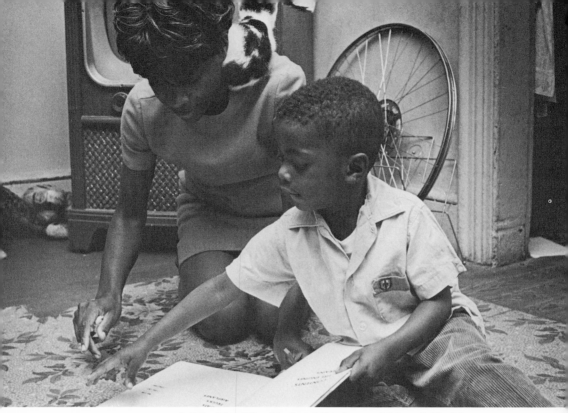

Calvin Nophlin, National Institute of Mental Health

Young children raised their IQ scores dramatically in a project sponsored by the National Institute of Mental Health. Tutors helped stimulate the youngsters' curiosity by reading to them, playing with them, and taking them on walks and trips.

group received no special attention, while the other met with tutors every day. Since the youngsters were too small for formal schooling, the tutors simply played with them, talked to them, read to them, and took them on walks and trips. They helped stimulate the youngsters to see, hear, and feel the world around them.

When the children reached the age of three, they were given intelligence tests. The tutored youngsters scored an average IQ of 106, which is above normal, while the untutored group scored an average of 89—well below normal.

The Swiss psychologist Jean Piaget has spent his life studying mental development in children. According to Piaget, the more new things a child has seen and heard, the more he wants to see and hear. The greater variety of experiences he has had, the greater is his ability to deal with new experiences.

The brain's only contact with the outside world comes through the body's senses—through the eyes, ears, nose, and tongue, and through nerve endings in the skin which register touch, pressure, heat, cold, and pain. Our sense organs are the gateways through which information from the outside world is channeled to the brain. They are the brain's only source of information about the world in which it must live and function.

CHAPTER 2

Tuning in on the World

A frog sits quietly at the edge of a pond, its bronze eyes bulging. Above the still water, dragonflies dart back and forth like miniature helicopters—dipping and hovering, occasionally landing on a lily pad or cattail reed. And in the tall grass nearby, mosquitoes hum.

Soon a ladybug appears on the scene. She wings her way low over the pond and lands on the bank where the frog waits motionless. The ladybug pauses, then begins to crawl past the frog. Suddenly the frog lunges forward, flicks out its sticky tongue, and swallows the ladybug in one gulp.

The frog's movement attracts the attention of a boy who is collecting specimens for his science class. He creeps up on the frog, raises his net, and starts to swing. Just then, the frog leaps into the safety of the water.

What signals made the frog react like this? How does a frog tell the difference between a ladybug it wants to eat and a boy it must escape from?

What the Frog's Eye Tells the Frog's Brain

A frog's eye, like all other sense organs, is a device for detecting signals from the world around. At the rear of a

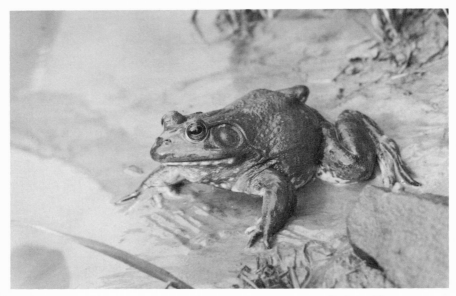

Robert Flanagan

Frog's-eye view: does the world look the same to a frog as it does to a human?

frog's eye is a membrane made up of tiny living cells called *neurons,* or nerve cells. Although these cells are too small to be seen without a microscope, they perform a vital and highly specialized task. Nerve cells in the frog's eye are sensitive to signals of reflected light. The cells convert light signals into faint electrical impulses which speed along nerve pathways to the frog's brain.

All sense organs, in animals and humans alike, work in essentially the same way. Each samples some part of the environment, then converts the signals to which it is sensitive into electrical nerve impulses. Every eye contains special light-sensitive nerve cells. Every ear has nerve cells that pick up vibrations of sound. The nose contains nerve cells that detect the chemicals of odor, while the tongue has nerve cells sensitive to the chemicals of taste. In the skin, millions of specialized nerve cells react to touch, pressure, heat, cold, and pain.

While some nerve cells pick up signals from the surrounding world, others specialize in transmitting that information to the brain. These cells make up the body's complex network of nerve pathways. The brain itself is an enormous cluster of specialized nerve cells that receive and interpret incoming information from the senses. Billions of nerve cells working together make up the body's nervous system.

Although nerve cells specialize in different tasks, they all have the same general design and follow the same plan of action. A nerve cell belonging to a frog is not much different from one belonging to a fish or a bird or a human. A typical nerve cell consists of a main cell body with long, thread-like fibers branching out from it in all directions. The main body of the cell is like a tiny living battery. Using a chemical fuel of sugar and oxygen, the cell is capable of generating a minute charge of electricity. As this electrical charge builds up, the cell "fires" and then recharges itself in a fraction of a second, so it is ready to "fire" again. Each discharge is a faint electrical impulse that travels away from the cell body through one of its thread-like fibers. Other nerve cells along the way act as relay stations, receiving the electrical impulse and passing it on.

The fiber that carries an impulse away from a "firing" nerve cell is called an *axon*. At the end of each axon, a tiny gap, or *synapse*, separates one nerve cell from another. When an electrical impulse reaches this gap, the nerve ending must secrete a temporary chemical bridge before the impulse can cross the gap and continue on to the next nerve fiber. This means that the impulse moves

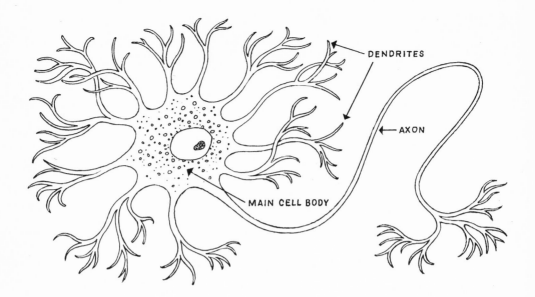

Typical nerve cell. Dendrites carry messages moving into the cell; axons carry messages away from the cell.

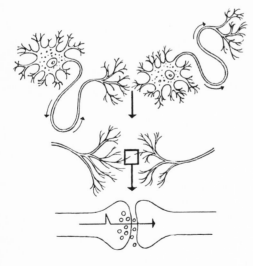

A synapse is the junction between two nerve cells. When an electrical impulse reaches the synapse, the nerve ending secretes a temporary chemical bridge so that the impulse can cross the gap.

Cross-section of a nerve. Each nerve consists of many nerve fibers bound together like wires in a cable.

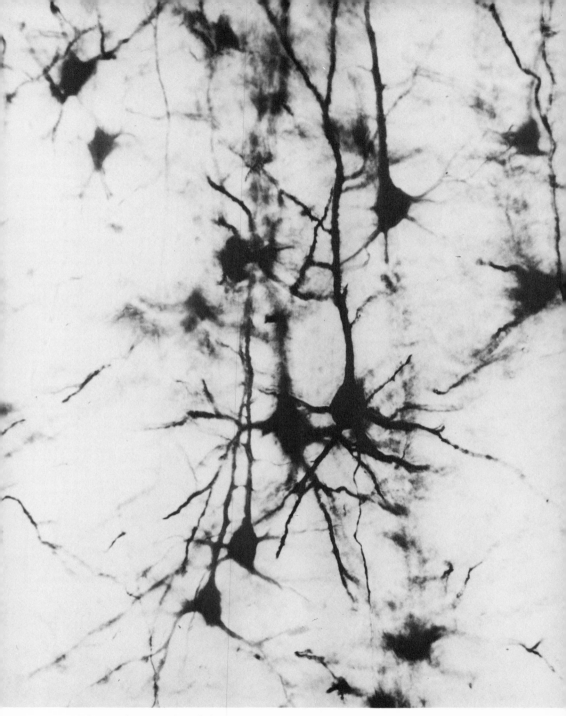

Photomicrograph of large nerve cells in the brain. A special staining method reveals the cell bodies and their projecting fibers. *Cover photo from* SCIENCE, *Vol. 144, 3 April 1964. Copyright* © *1964 by the American Association for the Advancement of Science.*

along step by step, in quick little spurts, like a spark traveling along the fuse of a firecracker. As it crosses the synaptic gap from one nerve cell to the next, each cell undergoes the same chemical and electrical changes and "fires" in turn.

The fibers that carry a nerve impulse toward the center of a neighboring cell are called *dendrites*. Nerve fibers are thus like one-way streets. Dendrites carry only those impulses moving into a cell, while axons carry impulses moving away from a cell. As an impulse travels through the nervous system from one cell to the next, it can move only in one direction. In order for an impulse to move in the opposite direction, it must travel through an entirely different set of nerve pathways.

What we usually call a "nerve" is actually a bundle of long, branching fibers from many nerve cells, bound together like wires in a cable. Nerves connect the brain to every part of the body.

A frog's eye, for example, is connected to its brain by the optic nerve. When the eye picks up light signals, electrical impulses travel through the optic nerve to a certain area of the brain, where the impulses are interpreted. The brain may then "fire" new impulses which travel along different nerve pathways to muscles in the frog's legs. As the muscles react, the frog leaps forward to capture a bug or to escape from danger.

But what does the frog actually see as it watches a bug crawling by or a boy with a net approaching? Does the world look the same to a frog as it does to a human?

At the Massachusetts Institute of Technology, a team of scientists headed by Dr. Jerome Y. Lettvin "listened in" on the electrical impulses traveling from a frog's eye to its brain. To begin with, Dr. Lettvin performed a minor operation. He removed a small section of skin and skull just behind the frog's eye, exposing the bundle of nerve fibers that make up the frog's optic nerve. Then, with the aid of a special microscope, he pushed tiny wire electrodes into the nerve fibers. The electrodes were connected to sensitive measuring instruments that could detect faint electrical impulses speeding to the frog's brain.

An electrode conducts electricity. The wire electrodes used by Dr. Lettvin were actually small enough to pierce microscopic nerve fibers without damaging them. Using this "wire-tapping" technique, Dr. Lettvin and his colleagues were able to listen in on the "line." The next step was to find out exactly when the frog's eye sends messages to the brain, and what it sends messages about.

After experimenting with many frogs, the M.I.T. scientists found that nerve cells in a frog's eye transmit four different kinds of information to the brain. Some cells detect contrast in the environment. They respond to all objects that are either lighter or darker than the background against which they appear. The only messages sent to the frog's brain by these nerve cells are information about the contrast of light and dark.

Other cells detect moving objects that come into view. The size or shape of the object makes little difference. Anything that moves across the frog's field of vision causes these nerve cells to respond. The faster the object moves, the more rapidly the cells "fire." If the object stops moving, the cells stop "firing."

A third group of cells reacts to any sudden decrease in

light, such as a shadow cast by a moving object. The ability to detect both falling shadows and quick movements can alert a frog to the approach of possible danger. If a boy sneaks up on a frog, casting a shadow, and begins to swing his net quickly, danger signals race to the frog's brain and the frog leaps to safety.

The nerve cells in the fourth group are the most interesting of all, for they are the "bug detectors" of the frog's eye. These cells respond only to small moving ob-

Electronic device "sees" like a frog. Built for research purposes, this machine utilizes six layers of photocells to duplicate the functions of a frog's retina. Output panel being held at left shows what the machine (or a frog) sees.

Courtesy of RCA

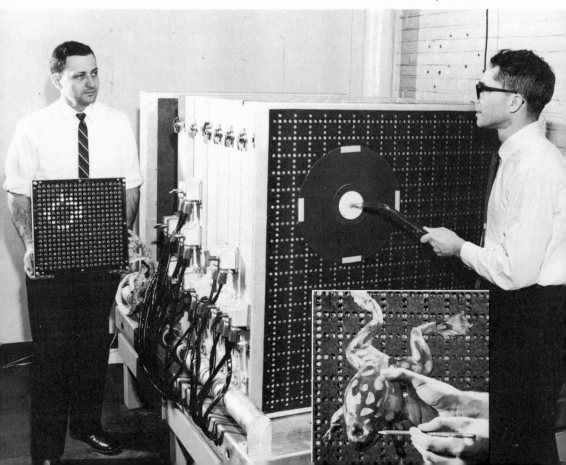

jects with curved surfaces. In the frog's natural environment, insects are about the only small moving objects with rounded edges. In the laboratory, however, a hungry frog will snap at pencil erasers, paper clips, or buttons that are tied to a string and dangled in front of its eyes. These objects must be made to move before the frog will respond. This explains why a frog surrounded by freshly killed but motionless insects will starve to death.

The brain can perceive only what the senses are able to detect. Although a frog is unable to see all the colors, forms, and textures that the human eye perceives, it survives quite well in its natural surroundings with its built-in bug detector and with its quick responses to falling shadows and sudden movements.

A frog's-eye view of the world is quite different from a man's-eye view. Like the frog, every living creature is limited in what it can see, hear, and feel by the kinds of information its senses are able to detect.

PROJECT

Do Frogs Prefer Blue?

Dr. W. R. A. Muntz, a scientist from England, first became interested in frog vision while working at Dr. Jerome Lettvin's laboratory at the Massachusetts Institute of Technology. Dr. Muntz discovered that a frog's eye is sensitive to certain colors. When tested in a special "jumping box" like the one shown on the next page, frogs seemed to prefer blue. Even when the other color used in the test was blue-green, frogs jumped through the pure blue window seventy-one percent of the time. Using microelectrode listening devices, Dr.

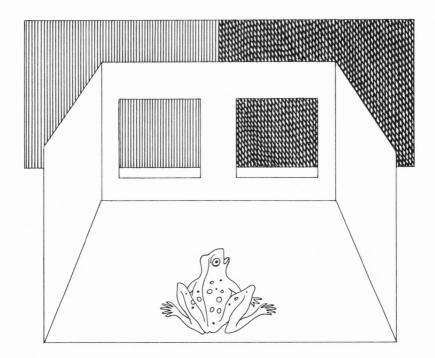

Muntz found that the color blue caused a burst of electrical activity in a frog's brain that lasted for several seconds. Green, yellow and red, on the other hand, produced only a few faint electrical impulses in the frog's brain.

Does a frog's preference for blue serve some useful function? Dr. Muntz believes that it does. Frogs live near the edges of ponds, in the grass and under trees. A frog may be surrounded by greenery and the pond itself may be hidden from sight. But in the direction of the water there is likely to be blue light reflected from the open sky over the pond. Even on a cloudy day, light over the pond would contain more blue and less green than light reflected from the vegetation surrounding the frog. It is quite possible, says Dr. Muntz, that sensitivity to blue light guides a frightened frog so that it leaps toward the water and escapes its enemies.

To test a frog's preference for blue:

1. Cut two windows side by side in a cardboard box, as shown above. A few inches behind the windows place construction paper backdrops of the colors you wish to test. Each backdrop must be brightly illuminated. Now place a frog in this "jumping box."

2. Keep a record of the number of times the frog jumps through each of the windows. You may have to prod your frog to make him jump.

3. After a few trials, switch the colored backdrops so that you can be sure the frog is responding to color and not just jumping in a particular direction. Does the frog's preference remain the same when the colors are switched?

4. Test a variety of colors. After many trials determine what percentage of the frog's responses were in the direction of blue backdrops. Does the frog's response to blue remain the same during each series of trials?

Signals from the Surrounding World

All living things are sensitive to the world around them. Plants respond to water, light, and chemicals in the soil, and some plants are sensitive to touch. Tiny microscopic creatures, whose bodies consist only of a single cell, are sensitive too. Paramecia, for example, will actively seek out darkness. If an aquarium containing these one-celled organisms is shaded so that one half is in light and the other half in darkness, they will gather on the dark side.

Paramecia are particularly sensitive to touch. If you

watch one of them under a microscope, you will see its slipper-shaped body darting quickly about—bumping into objects, backing away, then hurrying off in another direction.

Of course, one-celled organisms have no sense organs, no nervous systems, and no brains. They are limited in the information they can pick up from their environments just as they are limited in the kinds of responses they can make. Animals, whose bodies consist of many cells, are far more responsive because they possess special equipment for tuning in on the world. Even a primitive animal like the jellyfish is better informed about its surroundings than any one-celled organism. A jellyfish has

Paramecia as seen through a microscope.

Morty Segal

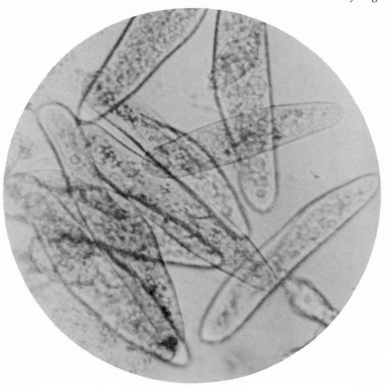

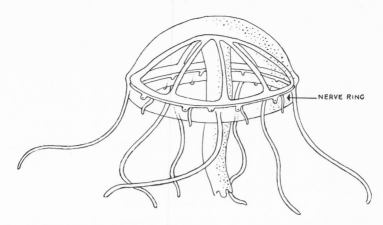

NERVE RING

Central nerve ring of a jellyfish. Electrical impulses travel around the nerve ring and then spread out to each tentacle.

no brain and no highly developed sense organs, but it does have a simple nervous system which permits the various parts of its body to work together as it swims through the ocean and captures food.

Scattered throughout the body of a jellyfish are nerve cells that specialize in the job of detection. Some of these cells can detect reflected light, but most of them are sensitive to touch. The touch-sensitive cells are especially numerous in the jellyfish's dangling tentacles. When a fish brushes against a tentacle, the touch-sensitive cells react. They fire electrical impulses which travel through the jellyfish's body.

The impulses follow a nerve pathway up the tentacle to a central nerve ring in the middle of the jellyfish's body. Moving around and around this central nerve ring, the impulses spread out to other parts of the body, causing muscles in each tentacle to contract, or tighten up. As this happens, the jellyfish entangles its victim, stings it to death, scoops it up, and stuffs it into its mouth.

Because the jellyfish has no brain to act as a command headquarters, it has no real control over its individual tentacles. It cannot move each tentacle separately, as a person can move each finger separately. If you were to touch one tentacle hard enough, all the tentacles would start moving. This muscular reaction is similar to a simple reflex in the human body. The tentacles move quite automatically—just as your leg jerks upward automatically when the doctor taps a nerve below your knee.

Compared with higher animals, a jellyfish has a poorly organized and extremely simple nervous system. Lacking even the beginnings of a brain to sort out incoming messages, this creature has no way of interpreting complex information from the outside world.

The Brain: From Worms to Man

Worms are the simplest animals to possess the beginnings of a brain. A flatworm has a small cluster of nerve cells in its head which act as a control center for the rest of its body. Extending from this primitive brain are two nerve cords which run down the flatworm's body from head to tail. Along the way, fibers branch out from the nerve cords, connecting each part of the flatworm's body with "headquarters" up front.

One kind of flatworm is called a planarian. Most people have never seen these creatures because they are so small, yet they are quite common in ponds, pools, and streams. Because of their tiny brains, they are able to organize information coming in from their senses and coordinate their body responses.

On top of its head, a planarian has two simple eyes. Since each eye contains only a few light-sensitive cells, the planarian cannot actually "see." But it can distinguish

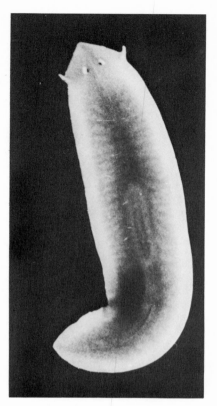
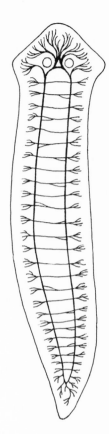

(Left) Enlarged planarian. Note the eye-spots and touch-knobs at the top of its head. (Right) Diagram of a planarian nervous system. A cluster of nerve cells in the head acts as a control center for the rest of the body.

between darkness and light, and it can even tell which direction the light is coming from. It also has knobs on either side of its head which are sensitive to touch, to water currents, and to certain chemicals, and which help the planarian detect the presence of food.

These sense organs transmit nerve impulses directly to the planarian's brain, which in turn sends impulses to the planarian's muscles. With its brain acting as command headquarters, the planarian is guided on its travels by the eyes and touch-knobs at the front end of its body. Crawling over rocks and plants, gliding through the water, it can turn purposefully in one direction or another—moving toward food, for instance, or toward a shady spot where it can hide. It has more control over its body than a jellyfish, and is more aware of changing conditions in its surroundings.

Many lower animals—those without backbones—have more complex brains than the planarian and more highly developed senses. Some mollusks, such as snails and slugs, have eyes on the end of retractable stalks that pull in like adjustable antennas on TV sets. While their eyes are still comparatively simple, these animals can detect shape and movement—which a planarian cannot.

Insects have more complex brains than mollusks and often possess remarkable sense organs. Many insects have excellent eyes, as anyone who has ever tried to swat a fly can testify. Bees can locate flowers by their color and can even detect ultraviolet rays of light which are beyond the range of human vision. Some insects also have finely tuned senses of taste and smell. Some male moths can detect the odor of a female from seven miles away.

An insect's brain is connected to a central nerve cord which runs along the insect's belly. In higher animals—those with backbones—the position of the central nerve cord is reversed. It runs along the back, protected by the bony tube of the spinal column, and is called the spinal cord. When we examine these higher animals—from fish to reptiles, birds, and mammals—we find that the brain becomes increasingly larger and the sense organs more

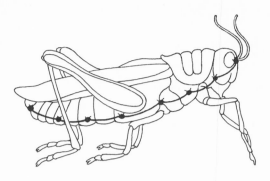

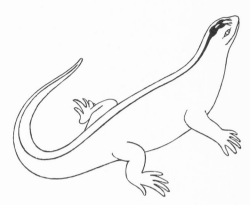

An insect has a central nerve cord running along its belly. Nerve clusters called *ganglia* are located in the head and at various points in the body.

A lizard has a well-developed brain and a spinal cord.

Enlarged head of a housefly. Many insects have excellent eyes.

A Shell photograph

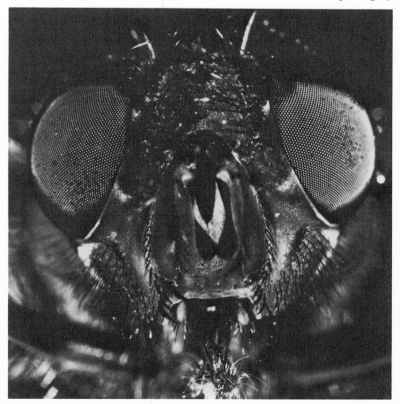

refined. Since these animals can pick up a greater variety of sights, sounds, and sensations from the world around them, they need more complex brains in order to process this information.

The kind of brain structure an animal has is related to the kind of life it leads, and to the senses that are most important to its survival. Fish have what some scientists have called a "nose brain." The largest and most prominent structures in a fish's brain are the *olfactory lobes,* which receive and process information about odors. Salmon have such an acute sense of smell, they are able to use their snouts as sensitive direction finders. When they return from their ocean migrations, they locate their home stream from among hundreds of others by zeroing in on its distinctive odor.

Birds, on the other hand, have little sense of smell. Instead, they rely heavily on their keen sense of vision. The olfactory lobes which handle "smell messages" are very small in a bird's brain, while large areas of its brain receive and process visual information. A bird can detect slight movements at great distances. Its eyes are sharp enough to spot tiny insects or seeds that it can eat. An insect-eating falcon can spot a dragonfly from half a mile away.

A world filled with meaningful odors.

Allan C. Bradbury

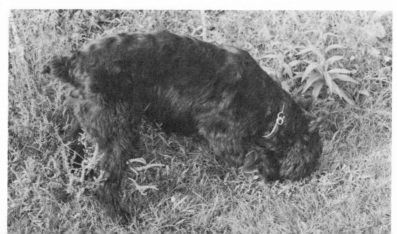

Like fish, many mammals are tuned into the world on channels of smell. To a dog or cat, a pig or a rat, scents convey more information than signals from any other senses. Meaningful odors guide these animals to their mates, warn them of their enemies, and help them find food. A hunting dog, sniffing through the woods, can detect the scent of a rabbit that may have hopped by half an hour before. The excited dog quickly picks up the trail and sets off in pursuit.

By stimulating a sense organ, and then noting which part of the brain becomes active with electrical discharges, scientists can measure the area of the brain that receives information from that particular sense. At Cambridge University in England, Dr. E. D. Adrian performed an experiment of this kind with a hedgehog, an animal that relies heavily on scent signals. A current of air was blown up into the hedgehog's nostrils. The odor of the air was so weak that the experimenters could not smell it at all, but the hedgehog certainly could. Electrical activity flared up in two-thirds of the surface of its brain.

Using similar techniques, scientists have measured the various areas of the human brain that receive messages from the senses. These receiving areas are called the brain's *projection areas*. Each sense organ is connected to its own projection area in the brain. In these areas, the electrical energy of nerve impulses is translated into meaningful sights, sounds, smells, tastes, and sensations.

A nerve impulse transmitted by the eye is essentially the same as an impulse transmitted by the ear or any other sense organ. The difference lies not in the impulse itself,

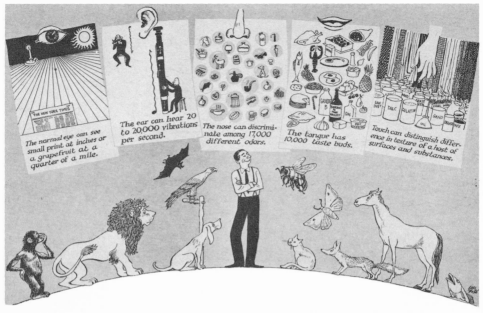

The normal eye can see small print at inches or a grapefruit at a quarter of a mile.

The ear can hear 20 to 20,000 vibrations per second.

The nose can discriminate among 17,000 different odors.

The tongue has 10,000 taste buds.

Touch can distinguish difference in texture of a host of surfaces and substances.

Drawing by Carl Rose

Human senses rank high when compared with the senses of animals.

but in the area of the brain that receives it. When injury or disease destroys one of these projection areas, the individual can no longer make use of the nerve impulses sent to that area. If the visual projection areas of a person's brain are destroyed, for example, he will suffer from a condition known as "mind blindness." Though he may have perfectly good eyes, he will not be able to see.

It is not the eye, then, that sees, nor the ear that hears, but the *brain*. If nerves from your eyes could be connected to the sound-receiving areas of your brain, and nerves from your ears connected to the visual-receiving areas, you would actually be able to see sounds and hear reflected light. Imagine a musician with his "wires crossed" in this way. If he were a guitarist, he might hear fantastic sounds whenever he looked at his instrument, and he might see visions when he plucked its strings. What a strange world it would be if our ears detected shapes and splashes of color, while our eyes opened each morning to a symphony of sound.

Designed for a medical convention, this complex assembly of disks and cables represents a human brain and its outlying sense organs. When the eyes (small disks at lower center) see an object, electrical messages flash along a cable to the consciousness screen (top center), where the image is projected.

Courtesy of The Upjohn Company, Kalamazoo, Mich. and the Cleveland Health Museum

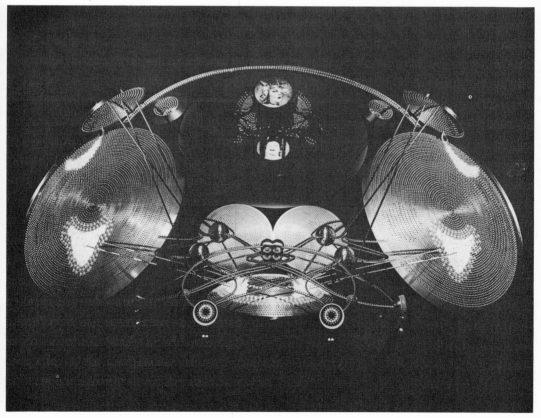

CHAPTER *3*

Mapping the Brain

The human brain is not much bigger than a grapefruit. It weighs about three pounds. Crammed into the bony hollow of the skull, surrounded and cushioned by a shock-absorbing fluid, it looks like a wrinkled glob of pinkish-gray jelly. Yet the brain contains roughly 12 billion nerve cells, and is alive with the electricity of consciousness.

This compact package of living nerve tissue is the most intricate, complex, and mysterious structure on earth. Scientists have probed its depths and mapped its surface inch by inch, but they have not yet discovered all its secrets. Even so, we know far more about the brain today than ever before in human history. Our ancestors knew practically nothing at all about the moist, spongy organ that controlled their thoughts, their passions, and their every movement.

The ancient Greeks didn't even have a name for the brain. To them it was simply "the thing in the head." They believed that thinking took place just above the midriff, while feelings originated just below it. Even today we reflect these early beliefs in our everyday speech. We still speak of "knowing in our hearts" or "believing deep inside."

If the Greeks thought that the center of our mental and

emotional lives was in the middle of the body, then what purpose did they think that "thing in the head" served? According to the Greek philosopher Aristotle, the brain was merely an air-conditioning device, designed by nature to cool overheated blood.

It is easy enough to understand why the ancients misunderstood the significance of the brain. After all, the brain hides silently behind the skull. We can't feel it. We aren't even aware of it. On the other hand, thoughts and feelings can provoke a variety of noticeable sensations throughout the body's mid-section. When you feel strongly about something, your heart beats faster. Fear or rage can make your heart pound, while the unexpected can cause it to "skip a beat." An unpleasant thought can "turn your stomach." The sudden realization that you have forgotten something can result in a "sinking feeling." Today we know that thoughts and emotions actually

Human brain as seen from the top: the most complex and mysterious structure on earth.

Rhode Island Hospital

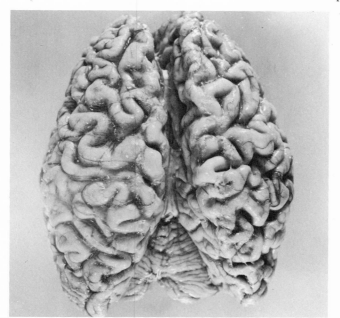

originate in the brain, and that the brain in turn affects the rest of the body. But the ancients had no way of knowing this.

Although most men in the ancient world failed to grasp the true importance of the brain, there were some exceptions. The Greek physician Hippocrates, who lived about the same time as Aristotle, had this to say about the human brain:

> "Men ought to know that from nothing else but the 'brain' come joys, delights, laughter . . . sorrows, grief, despondence. . . . And by the 'brain' in a special manner we acquire wisdom and knowlegde, and see and hear. . . . And by this same organ we become mad and delirious, and fears and terrors assail us, some by night and some by day."

Despite this perceptive guess, few men of the time agreed with Hippocrates. In fact, more than 2000 years were to pass before scientists began to discover that the Greek physician had spoken the truth.

Discovery of the Brain

About 300 years ago, an English doctor named Thomas Willis made a discovery that helped set the stage for modern brain research. At the time, medical science was breaking away from many mistaken notions of the past. Throughout Europe, physicians and scientists were charting and studying the body's muscles, blood vessels, and internal organs. Dr. Willis was particularly interested in the nerves. Since nerves are actually bundles of nerve

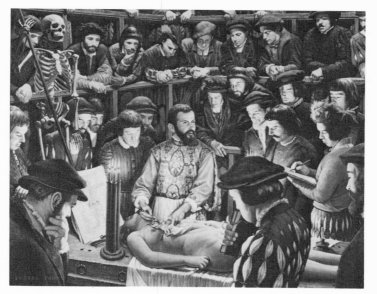

Throughout Europe, physicians were studying the body's muscles, blood vessels, nerves, and internal organs. This painting depicts Andreas Vesalius of Brussels, the first great teacher of anatomy from natural observations. As Professor of Anatomy at the University of Padua during the 16th century, Vesalius made many important discoveries about the human body.

fibers bound together, many of them are visible to the naked eye. Some nerves extend three feet or more through the body.

By tracing the paths of the body's chief nerves, Willis found that they all led to one place: the brain. He reasoned that if the brain was connected to the nerves, and the nerves branched out to all parts of the body, then the body and brain must be in close communication.

A century later, during the 1700's, scientists gained a better understanding of what nerves do and why they are so important. In Switzerland, Dr. Albrecht von Haller discovered that some nerves control the body's muscles. By stimulating a nerve leading to a muscle, he was able

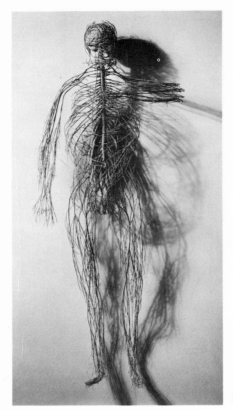

Courtesy of
The American Museum of
Natural History
Depiction in wire of the human nervous system.

to make that muscle contract, or tighten up. He then discovered that other nerves carry sensations, such as pressure or pain. If he cut a nerve leading to the skin, that particular section of skin would lose all feeling.

Von Haller believed that all the nerves meet in the middle of the brain. After years of experimentation, he suggested that the brain is the master control center of the nervous system; it receives messages from the senses by means of the *sensory nerves;* after interpreting these messages, the brain transmits instructions to the muscles by means of the *motor nerves.*

Other scientists, meanwhile, had been busy exploring the ridges and valleys on the brain's outer surface, and the strange bulges and chambers hidden below. Gradually, maps were drawn up showing the various regions of the brain's geography. In time, brain maps became more accurate and detailed. Almost from the beginning, however, pioneering brain researchers were able to identify the chief physical features of the human brain.

They found that the brain emerges from the spinal cord like a flower bursting from its stem. As the spinal cord enters the base of the skull, it widens and then bulges to form the *brainstem*. In the human body, the brainstem is about three inches long. Resting on top of it are two small structures called the *thalamus* and *hypothalamus*. The word "thalamus" means "inner chamber," while the prefix "hypo" means "below." Each of these structures lies hidden near the center of the head.

Overhanging these lower regions of the brain, and completely covering them, is the bulging, deeply wrinkled *cerebrum*. This is by far the largest and most prominent part of the human brain. It fills the whole upper portion of the skull, dominating the areas below. The cerebrum is divided into two halves, or hemispheres. Each cerebral hemisphere occupies one side of the skull.

The outer surface of the cerebrum is called the *cerebral cortex*, which means "brain bark." The cortex covers the cerebrum as bark covers a tree. However, only about one-third of the cortex is actually visible on the brain's surface. The rest is concealed by deep crevices and folds, called convolutions. If all these convolutions were smoothed out, the cortex would take up as much space as a newspaper page and would not fit inside the skull. We know today that the cortex is made up largely of

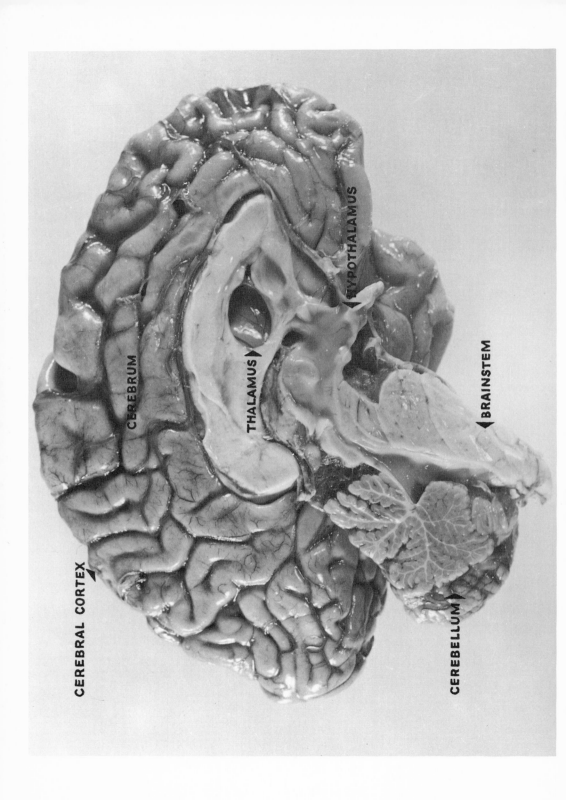

pinkish-gray nerve cell bodies. Beneath this "gray matter," the rest of the cerebrum consists mainly of long white nerve fibers branching out from the cell bodies above.

Tucked away at the base of the skull beneath the cerebrum is another important part of the brain—the *cerebellum*. Like the massive cerebrum that looms above it, the cerebellum is divided into two hemispheres and is tightly folded. Though it makes up ten percent of the brain's mass, it fits into a very small area. In fact, the word "cerebellum" means "little brain."

Early brain mappers could see that the human brain is divided into several distinct regions. But they did not yet realize that each region performs its own specialized functions.

Geography of the Brain

In 1861, a French surgeon named Pierre Broca conducted an autopsy on the body of a former patient. Before his death, the patient had lost the ability to speak. Dr. Broca examined the outer surface of this man's brain, searching for some sign of damage. The right side of the brain appeared to be normal. But a small area on the left side was visibly damaged. Was this the area of the brain that controls our ability to speak? Were other areas in charge of other physical functions?

Broca's discovery was quickly followed up by Dr. Hughlings Jackson, an English physician. He examined the brains of many former patients who, before their deaths, had lost the ability to use some part of their bodies. Like Broca before him, Jackson found that his patients had suffered visible brain damage. The damaged areas were apparently connected to the parts of the body that had stopped functioning. Gradually, Jackson was able to identify in a general way areas of the brain that seemed to be in charge of the body's muscles and sense organs.

Soon afterwards, Jackson's findings were verified by two German researchers, Gustav Fritsch and Eduard Hitzig, who began to explore the brain with a new tool: electricity. Scientists knew by now that messages traveling through the nerves are electrical in nature. Would it be possible to create artificial nerve messages by stimulating the brain with electricity?

Working in their Berlin laboratory, Fritsch and Hitzig applied weak electric currents to the exposed brain tissue of experimental dogs. During these experiments the dogs slept soundly under strong anesthetics, yet they still responded to electrical stimulation of their brains. Fritsch and Hitzig found that by stimulating different points on the outer surface of a dog's brain, they could make the sleeping dog move its paw, lift its leg, wag its tail, twitch its ears, turn its head, blink its eyes, and so on. When a specific point on the left side of the brain was stimulated, the dog would automatically move its right forepaw. When the corresponding point on the right side of the brain was stimulated, the dog would move its left forepaw. In this way, the German scientists demonstrated that nerves extending from the right cerebral hemisphere lead to the left side of the body, while nerves extending from the left cerebral hemisphere lead to the right side of the body.

By means of a weak electric current, it was possible to

turn behavior on and off. The current had the same effect as if brain cells in the stimulated area had "fired" electrical impulses on their own. With this dramatic new technique, called Electrical Stimulation of the Brain, or ESB, researchers began to explore the brains of a wide variety of experimental animals.

Exploration of the human brain was more difficult. Humans could not be subjected to the same kind of experiments that revealed so much about the brains of

Brain surgery has contributed greatly to our knowledge of the brain's specialized functions. This operation is being performed by a team of neurosurgeons from the National Institute of Neurological Diseases and Stroke.

Roy Perry, National Institutes of Health

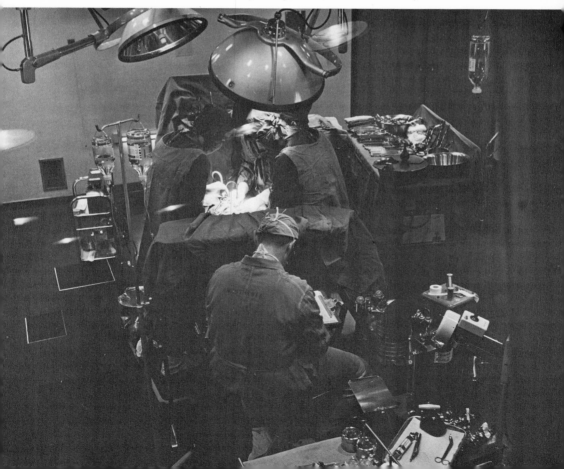

animals. Yet information was gradually accumulated. Brain injuries sustained during war or accident provided medical science with thousands of case studies. Surgery contributed greatly to our knowledge of the brain's specialized functions. During operations for the removal of tumors and diseased brain tissue, it was often possible to verify the findings that had been made in animal experiments.

An important contribution to our understanding of the human brain was made during the 1940's by Dr. Wilder Penfield, a surgeon and nerve specialist at Canada's Montreal Neurological Institute. During hundreds of brain operations, Dr. Penfield used a tiny electric needle to explore the cerebral cortex—the outer covering of the brain. Since there are no pain-sensing nerves in the brain, many brain operations can be performed with a local anesthetic that deadens only a small section of the skull. After the anesthetic is applied, the doctor cuts out an opening in the skull, giving access to the brain. As the operation proceeds, the patient remains fully conscious and can tell the doctor what he is thinking and feeling.

Using this technique over a period of many years, Dr. Penfield was able to map large areas of the brain's outer surface. He gradually identified those areas of the cerebral cortex that control muscular movement and those that receive messages from the senses.

Motor and sensory areas of the human brain.

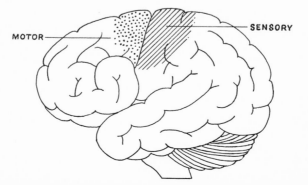

MOTOR   SENSORY

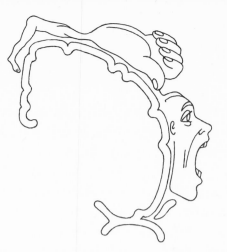

This diagram of a misshapen little man, called the "motor homunculus," was used by Dr. Wilder Penfield to show the amount of brain tissue that controls muscles in each part of the body. More brain tissue is devoted to the hand than the foot, for example, because the hand has more muscles. Dr. Penfield mapped the muscle-controlling points of the cortex during hundreds of brain operations.

The muscle-controlling or *motor area* forms a wide band across the top of the brain. Each group of voluntary muscles in the body has a corresponding "control point" somewhere in this motor area. Using his electric probe, Dr. Penfield could make a patient move the little finger of his left hand by stimulating a specific control point on the right side of the motor area. By stimulating other specific control points, he could make the patient bend his elbow, twist his neck, open his mouth, or move any other group of muscles.

Dr. Penfield found that the amount of brain surface controlling a certain part of the body depends on how much that part of the body is used. For example, the section of the brain that controls hand muscles is much larger than the section that controls foot muscles. Since the hand is used more than the foot, it has a larger portion of the brain devoted to it. You can move each of your fingers separately, enabling you to handle tools and other objects, but you cannot move your toes separately. For the same reason, the section of the brain that controls the mouth is larger than the sections that control all the other facial muscles. Since we use our mouths to form words, we must be able to move our tongues and lips in many different ways. Try moving your lips about for a moment. Now try moving the muscles in the rest of your face.

Directly behind the motor area, Dr. Penfield identified another wide band running across the top of the brain. This *sensory area* receives messages from millions of nerve endings in the skin and interprets them as various degrees of pressure, pain, heat, and cold. If you burn the little finger of your right hand, nerve impulses travel to a specific point in the sensory area, allowing you to identify the kind of pain and to pinpoint its exact location. If an ant crawls up your leg, or a friend taps you on the shoulder, or a raindrop falls on your head, the sensory area of your brain tells you exactly what part of your body is being touched. When Dr. Penfield moved his electric probe across this area of the brain, the patient felt tingling sensations in each successive part of his body.

Behind and below the sensory area, other specialized areas of the cerebral cortex receive nerve impulses coming from the eyes, the ears, and the nose. We see with the back part of our brains, hear with the side parts, and smell with the bottom parts. These areas can also be stimulated with an electric probe. If the visual area at the back of the brain is stimulated, the patient sees flashes of light. If the auditory areas on either side of the brain are stimulated, the patient hears bursts of sound, even though the room is completely silent.

In the human brain, only about one-fourth of the cortex seems to be directly in charge of the muscles and sense organs. What about the other three-fourths? These areas do not seem to respond when they are stimulated by an electric probe. For this reason they were originally called "silent areas." Today, however, they are known as the brain's *association areas* because they apparently bring together different kinds of information coming from all the senses. If you pick up an orange, for instance, you feel the orange with one part of your brain, see it with another part, and perhaps smell it with still another part. The association areas of the cortex make it possible for you

Compare the brains. As we examine the higher animals—from fish to amphibians, reptiles, birds, and mammals—we find that the brain increases in size and complexity.

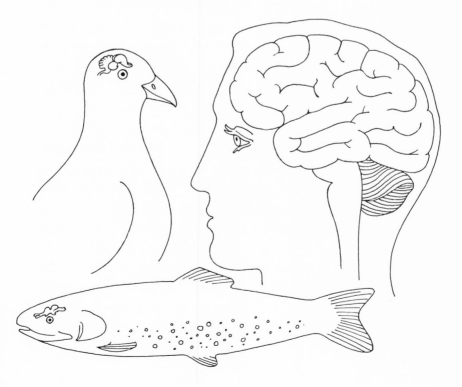

to fit these separate impressions together like pieces of a jigsaw puzzle, forming a meaningful picture of the orange. Scientists believe that the association areas are also concerned with memory, learning, and thinking—enabling you to recognize the orange as something good to eat, to peel it, and to bite into it.

The cerebral cortex, with its vast association areas, forms the outer crust of the massive human cerebrum. This part of the brain marks one of the chief differences between man and beast. In animals such as fish and frogs, the cerebrum has just begun to develop and no cortex or outer bark of cells is present. Among reptiles and birds, the cerebrum increases in size and shows the beginnings of a cortex. Among mammals, the cerebrum is the most prominent part of the brain. It reaches its highest development in humans, packing the skull and completely covering the lower, more primitive parts of the brain. Hidden deep beneath this bulging, wrinkled structure are the areas of the brain that control basic drives such as hunger and thirst, and powerful emotions such as fear, rage, and pleasure.

Probing the Depths of Emotion

One of the first men to explore the inner recesses of the brain was Dr. Walter R. Hess, a physiologist at the University of Zurich in Switzerland. His tools of exploration were needle-like tubes that carried a weak electric current. By inserting these tubes deeply into the brains of experimental animals, Hess was able to stimulate the *limbic system,* which is tucked away beneath the bulging mass of the cerebrum and which includes parts of the thalamus

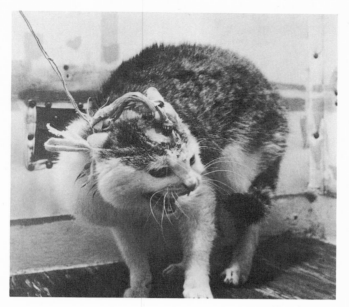

Probing the depths of emotion: while electrical stimulation of the brain is completely painless, it can trigger a variety of powerful emotions. This cat has electrodes implanted in a certain area of its hypothalamus, deep inside the brain. As a weak electric current flows into this area, the cat hisses and claws, displaying violent anger. When the current is shut off, the cat again becomes calm and affectionate.

and hypothalamus. The limbic system is one of the oldest and most primitive areas of the brain to develop in higher animals.

As Hess probed cautiously into this ancient "emotional brain," he made one startling discovery after another. By stimulating a certain section of the hypothalamus, for example, he found he could turn friendly cats into hissing, clawing bundles of fury. With tails puffed out, fur standing on end, and eyes searching frantically about the laboratory, the cats were ready to attack anything in sight, including the experimenters. But as soon as the electric current was switched off, their anger subsided. Once again, they became as friendly as ever.

By stimulating another section of the hypothalamus, Hess found that he could "turn on" a cat's hunger drive, even though the cat had already gorged itself with food. No matter how much a cat had already eaten, it would continue to stuff itself until Hess turned off the electric current that was stimulating the appetite-control area of its brain. If no food was available when its hunger drive was turned on, the cat would attempt to eat its food tray or the bars of its cage.

With his electrified tubes, Hess was able to trigger not only hunger and rage, but also thirst, fatigue, anxiety, and fear. His pioneering experiments during the 1930's later earned him a Nobel Prize. Since then, other brain researchers have continued his exploration of the brain's interior and have refined his methods.

When an animal is prepared for deep brain stimulation, it is first put to sleep with an anesthetic. During the

A special measuring device, called a stereotaxic apparatus, is used to guide a hair-thin silver electrode to a selected site within the brain. When the experimental animal awakens, it will not be aware of the implanted electrode, since the brain itself has no feeling.

Tom Leyden

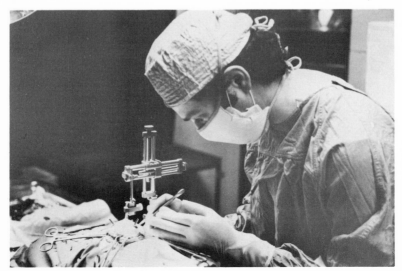

delicate operation that follows, the animal's head is held firmly in place by the metal frame of a special measuring device, called a stereotaxic apparatus. The experimenter lowers a high-speed drill into position, and in an instant bores a tiny hole through the skull. Then, with the aid of the stereotaxic apparatus, he slowly drives a silver wire thinner than a human hair into the soft brain tissue. Carefully, he guides the wire electrode to a selected point within the brain. Here it will remain like an artificial nerve, ready to carry electric impulses to the region where it is lodged. Finally, the experimenter connects the outer end of the wire electrode to a small plastic socket, which he cements to the animal's skull. By applying a mild electric current to this socket, he can now stimulate the area of the brain where the silver wire is implanted.

When the animal awakens, it will not be aware of the electrode within its brain, for the brain itself has no feeling. Animals have remained perfectly healthy through hundreds of brain stimulation experiments. They sometimes live for many years with plastic sockets cemented to their skulls and wire electrodes implanted in their brains.

Occasionally, however, an electrode may miss its mark. One such accident resulted in an unexpected discovery about the brain. At McGill University in Canada during the 1950's, Dr. James Olds was investigating the functions of the brainstem. He had implanted electrodes in the brainstems of several laboratory rats. Sockets in the rats' skulls were connected to a power source by means of long wire cords, which permitted the rats to move freely about their cages. When a rat entered a certain corner of its cage, a mild electric current was sent to its brainstem. Al-

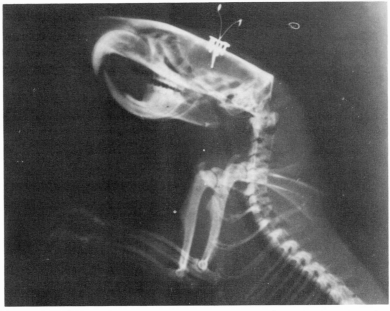

This X-ray photograph shows electrodes implanted in the brain of a laboratory rat. The electrodes are attached to a plastic socket screwed into the skull. They can be used to transmit electrical stimulation to the brain or to record electrical impulses generated by the brain.

though the current caused no pain, it did cause an unpleasant sensation. The rats quickly learned to avoid this sensation by staying away from that corner of the cage.

One rat behaved strangely, however. Instead of avoiding the corner of the cage where it received electrical brain stimulation, the rat refused to leave that corner. If it was picked up and removed to an opposite corner of its cage, it would run back to the stimulation corner as if asking for more.

This behavior was not what Dr. Olds had expected. An examination revealed that the electrode had somehow veered off course. Instead of going directly to the brainstem as intended, it had entered the main bundle of nerve fibers that ties together the limbic system. Here, in the depths of the old emotional brain, Dr. Olds had accidentally discovered what seemed to be a "pleasure center."

Since the rat seemed to enjoy electrical discharges in this area of its brain, Dr. Olds decided to see what would happen if the rat were allowed to control its own brain stimulation. He installed a lever in the rat's cage. The lever was hooked up to a battery, which was connected to the electrode in the rat's brain. Before long, the rat learned to press the lever with its paw. Each time it did so, it delivered an electric current to its brain and experienced a brief moment of pleasurable stimulation. Soon the animal was pressing the lever as fast as it could. It gave up food, water, and even sleep in order to stay close beside the lever and keep on pressing it.

(Left) A laboratory rat seeks to stimulate the "pleasure center" of its brain as it places its paw on the lever. (Right) When the rat pushes the lever, a weak electric current flows into its brain. The current lasts less than a second, and the rat must push the lever again to renew the stimulation. Some animals pressed pleasure levers in their cages as often as 8000 times an hour.

Dr. James Olds

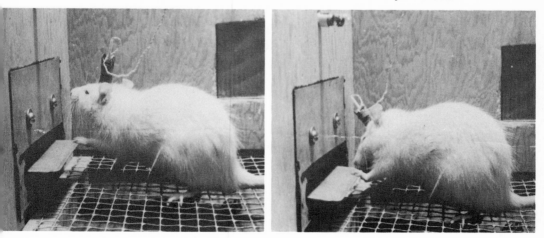

Other rats behaved the same way when wire electrodes were deliberately implanted in the pleasure centers of their brains. Some of them pressed levers in their cages at the phenomenal rate of 8000 times an hour. Many of these rats would not stop their lever pressing until they dropped from exhaustion. And rats kept on a starvation diet for ten days would, if given the chance, select brain stimulation over food.

Since Dr. Olds' accidental discovery, much progress has been made in mapping pleasure centers in the brains of cats, dogs, monkeys, apes, dolphins, and other animals. Of course, an animal cannot tell the experimenter exactly how it feels when the pleasure centers of its brain are being stimulated. However, human patients undergoing brain operations have experienced similar stimulation. They have reported marvelous sensations of "well-being," of "happiness," and of generally "feeling good."

Deep brain stimulation has provided valuable insights into the emotional lives of both animals and humans. And yet the hidden regions of the brain, with their incredibly complex networks of interlocking nerve connections, are the most difficult to explore. One difficulty is that certain powerful feelings seem to arise in more than one area of the emotional brain. Scientists can provoke fighting rage in a laboratory monkey by stimulating any one of at least five separate structures in the monkey's inner brain. The brain also contains several separate but closely related pleasure-producing sites. In fact, the exact location of these pleasure centers differs somewhat in different kinds of animals.

Another difficulty in deep brain stimulation is that

tiny, hard-to-reach structures, such as the hypothalamus, somehow perform a staggering variety of tasks. The hypothalamus is no bigger than a prune, and it accounts for only three-hundredths of the brain's total weight. Even so, it is the control center for some of our most powerful emotions and drives. It not only contains one of the brain's chief pleasure centers, but also contributes to feelings of fear and rage. In addition to this, the hypothalamus regulates the body's temperature and activates certain behavior necessary for survival, such as eating, drinking, sleeping, mating, fighting, and fleeing. When we feel threatened, it mobilizes our bodies for self defense. The pounding heart, sweaty palms, and dry mouth of intense emotion are all controlled by the tiny hypothalamus.

Another vital area of the hidden brain is the thalamus, or "inner chamber," which lies just above the hypothalamus. It is here that we first become vaguely aware of sensations such as pressure, pain, heat, and cold. However, the thalamus cannot determine exactly where in the body these sensations originate. And it cannot tell exactly what causes them. If you step on a tack, the thalamus

Buried deep within the brain, the tiny thalamus and hypothalamus control a variety of emotions, drives, and vital physical functions.

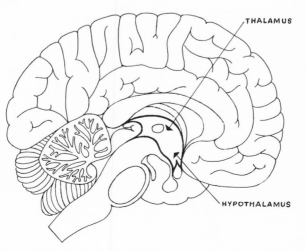

THALAMUS

HYPOTHALAMUS

registers a generalized feeling of pain somewhere in the lower part of your leg. But before you actually realize that the pain is in the sole of your foot, and that it was caused by a pointed object, nerve impulses must be transmitted from the thalamus to the sensory area of the cerebral cortex, the thinking part of the brain. The thalamus thus serves as a crucial relay station where nerve impulses are crudely interpreted and sorted before being sent on to the cortex above. Among its other functions, the thalamus regulates our feelings of discomfort and well-being, and our cycles of wakefulness and sleep.

Below the thalamus and hypothalamus lies the brainstem, which connects the brain to the spinal cord. One specialized area of the brainstem, the *medulla,* regulates breathing, swallowing, digestion, heartbeat, and other automatic physical functions. The brainstem is also a busy crossroads for nerve impulses speeding back and forth between the spinal cord and the higher centers of the brain.

Running through the brainstem is a collection of nerve cells called the *reticular formation.* Reticular means "net-

The reticular formation regulates our level of attention.

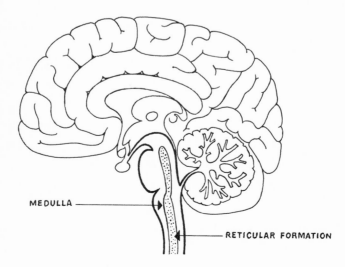

MEDULLA

RETICULAR FORMATION

like," and this closely woven network of nerves has received considerable attention in recent years. Brain researchers have discovered that the reticular formation acts as a kind of filter. It determines which impulses entering the brainstem will receive the attention of higher brain centers. We are constantly bombarded with sensations coming from both inside and outside our bodies. If you stop to think about it, you can feel the pressure of your clothes against your body, your tongue against your mouth, your fingers touching the pages of this book; perhaps you can hear the ticking of a clock, a radio playing in another room, the sounds of traffic on the street outside. Every living moment, even during sleep, millions of nerve impulses race through the spinal cord on their way to the brain. If all these impulses reached the upper regions of the brain, it would be overwhelmed. The reticular formation censors this incoming information. It regulates our level of attention, enabling us to concentrate on some signals from the surrounding world, and to ignore others.

Hidden away at the back of the head is one other specialized brain structure—the cerebellum, or "little brain." This organ directs no specific body function. Instead, it coordinates messages coming from other parts of the brain, acting as a mediator between them and the body. The cerebellum seems to have a collection of information about the body; it seems to know what each part of the body is doing at any given time—which muscles are in action and which are relaxed. In fact, the cerebellum works in close cooperation with the motor area on top of the brain. The motor area enables us to direct the movements of our voluntary muscles, while the

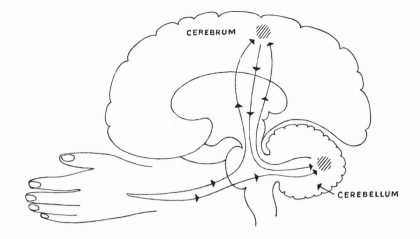

The cerebellum coordinates messages speeding back and forth between the muscle-controlling area of the cortex and various parts of the body.

Guided by the cooperative action of the brain, 32 muscles in each hand work smoothly and efficiently together.

Allan C. Bradbury

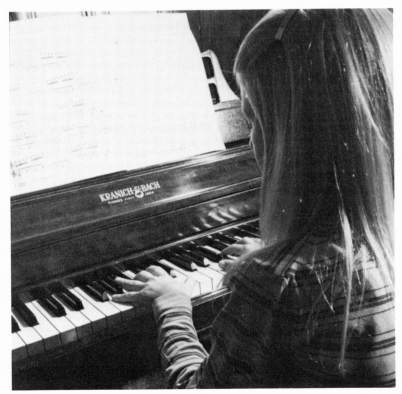

cerebellum actually controls the muscular movements involved. If you sit down to play the piano, the motor area of your brain makes it possible for you to consciously move your hands. But it is the cerebellum that unconsciously mobilizes the thirty-two separate muscles in each hand, coordinating their movements smoothly and efficiently without you having to think about them.

Each part of the brain, then, performs certain highly specialized tasks. However, billions of crisscrossing communication lines connect one part of the brain with another. As a result, complex behavior depends on the cooperative action of the brain as a whole.

The wrinkled cerebrum that fills our skulls controls our conscious activities. It interprets messages from our senses, and directs the movements of our bodies. It allows us to make meaningful associations, to remember, to think, and to plan. Yet this "knowing" part of the brain depends on information supplied by the more primitive regions below. It acts as a command headquarters, controlling and directing the drives and emotions that swell up from the lower regions of the brain. Without this emotional input, the cerebrum or "thinking brain" would be little more than a sophisticated computing mechanism. And without the cerebrum, we would be all feeling and no thought.

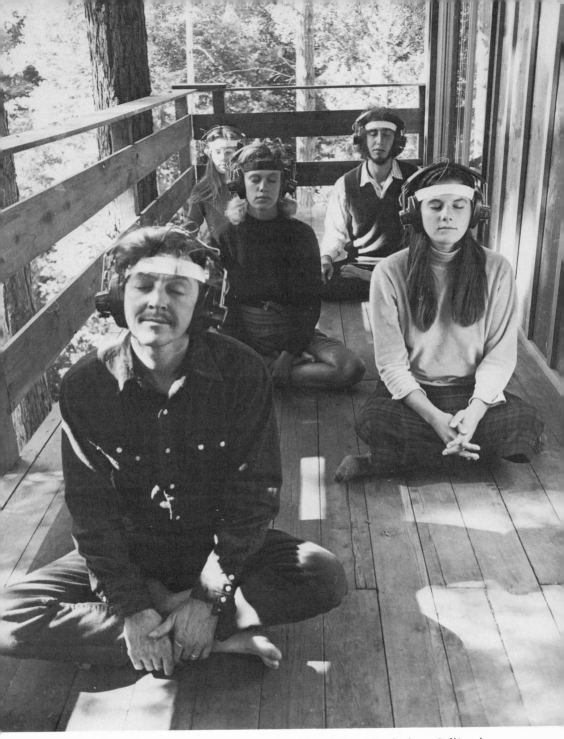

Listening for the magic tone.

CHAPTER *4*

Brain Waves

A group of young men and women sit quietly on the floor, legs crossed in the "lotus" position. Eyes closed, they listen intently for the sound of the magic tone from head-phones worn over their ears. One of the boys takes a deep breath and slowly begins to let it out. On his face he wears a look of serenity.

A girl in the group smiles softly to herself. She is getting an almost steady tone through her headphones. She had concentrated very hard learning how to produce this tone, and it tells her that her brain is emitting a steady stream of alpha waves. How wonderful, she thinks, to experience the thrill of controlling an inner state of feeling.

These young people are taking part in an unusual class. They are attempting to learn Yoga—a discipline that Hindu mystics have mastered for centuries. However, the young people are approaching Yoga through modern electronics. Their headphones are designed to put them in touch with their "inner selves," and perhaps open a way for them to extend the dimensions of their minds.

The technique they are using is called Bio-Feedback Training, or BFT. The special devices they wear on their heads are equipped to monitor waves of electrical energy generated by the brain. Each device consists of several metal electrodes held tightly in place against the scalp by a band worn around the head. Wires from the electrodes are connected to large earphones which convert certain brain waves into a musical tone. Using this tone as a guide, a person engaged in BFT can "turn on" those brain waves at will.

Scientists have identified four basic brain wave rhythms, which are labeled (from the Greek alphabet) *delta, theta, alpha,* and *beta.* Normally the human brain gives off a complex mixture of rhythms, yet certain kinds of brain waves seem to be associated with certain states of mind. A continuous discharge of alpha waves seems to reflect tranquillity and well-being. During profound meditation, Zen masters discharge an almost steady stream of alpha waves. In fact, scientists have found that experienced Zen meditators learn to exert amazing control not only over their brain waves, but over other body functions as well. By sheer force of will, they can slow down or speed up their heartbeats, raise or lower their blood pressure, reduce their body temperatures, and enter into deep states of trance. Before careful investigations proved otherwise, many scientists had considered these body functions forever beyond the reach of conscious control.

Learning body and mind control through traditional Yoga methods usually takes years of patient practice. But with electronic headsets and BFT, it now may be possible for an individual to control the state of his mind and body in a much shorter time. By concentrating on the musical tone that sounds when the brain produces alpha waves, the individual can learn to repeat that tone more and more often. After a few days of practice, many people find they can sustain for long periods both the musical tone and the tranquil mental state associated with alpha rhythms.

"All of this is very important to us," says Dr. Joseph Kamiya, a research specialist at the Langley Porter Neuropsychiatric Institute in San Francisco. "It shows that man is capable of achieving and controlling various states of consciousness that he is normally only vaguely aware of, if at all."

The Electrical Language of the Brain

For years, scientists have been interested in the electrical activity of the living brain. As millions of brain cells "fire" together, they produce rhythmic waves of electrical energy that pass continuously from the brain through the skull. Long before the invention of the new bio-feedback devices, hospitals and laboratories throughout the world were busy recording the brain-wave patterns of humans and a wide variety of animals.

Scientists normally "listen in" on the brain's electrical activity by pasting small metal strips to an individual's scalp. Each metal electrode can pick up faint electrical signals coming from inside the head. Wires connect the electrodes to a dial-studded machine which will convert the electrical signals into a written code. Stretched across the top of this machine is a wide strip of paper. And poised above the paper are eight or more pens, each connected to one of the electrodes on the subject's head.

When the machine is turned on, the strip of paper be-

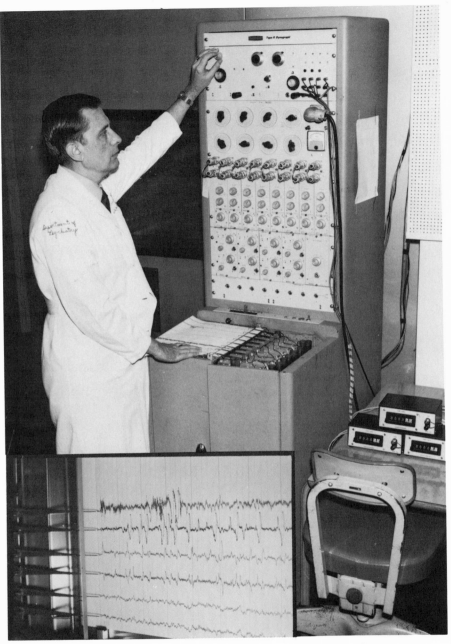

Dr. Stanley Krippner demonstrates a brain-wave recorder at Maimonides Medical Center in New York. (Inset) The electrical language of the brain. *James E. Morriss*

gins to move slowly like a conveyer belt, and the pens jump into action. Dancing about, swinging back and forth, the pens etch wavy black lines on the moving paper. These lines reflect the brain's special electrical rhythms.

Even if a scientist has never met you, he can learn a great deal about you by interpreting the written record of your brain waves. He can tell if you were awake or asleep when your brain waves were recorded, if your mind was relaxed or if you were concentrating. Often he knows if you were excited, frustrated, angry, or calm. And he can discover clues to your personality and the way you think.

Some brain-wave rhythms produce lazy, wobbly lines on a moving strip of paper. Others produce sharply angled lines. All of these lines together express the "work habits" of brain cells during normal everyday life. They also give warning if something goes wrong deep inside the brain. As a result, doctors can use brain-wave recordings as tools to diagnose brain diseases and to locate damaged tissue and tumors.

In order to record brain-wave rhythms, scientists must use sensitive electronic equipment. This equipment is needed to amplify, or strengthen, the weak electrical signals that pass through the thick shield of the skull. A single electrode pasted to the scalp may record a mere five-millionths of a volt. It would take perhaps 60 thousand scalps together to supply enough power to light a flashlight. A modern brain-wave recorder can amplify the brain's electrical activity a million times or more.

Today, brain-wave studies occupy a specialized branch of science called *electroencephalography,* which means

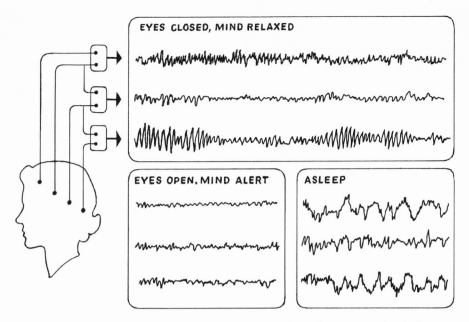

EYES CLOSED, MIND RELAXED

EYES OPEN, MIND ALERT

ASLEEP

Brain-wave recordings reveal a person's changing state of mind.

"electric brain writing." A brain-wave recording is called an *electroencephalogram,* or *EEG* for short.

When you first examine the up-and-down lines of an EEG, they seem to have about as much meaning as Arabic script would have for an American child. But to the brain-wave specialist, these lines have great significance. A certain change in a person's brain-wave pattern may mean that he has just opened his eyes. Other changes may indicate that he has seen a light go on, or heard a voice, or felt someone tap him on the shoulder. Each experience leaves its distinctive imprint in the lines of an EEG.

Thoughts and emotions also cause changes in the electrical activity of the brain. An EEG can reveal such aspects of a person's mental state as attentiveness and inattentiveness, certainty and uncertainty.

At Columbia University in New York City, Dr. Samuel Sutton demonstrated how brain waves can reflect changing states of mind. A woman sat in a dark, quiet room. Electrodes pasted to her scalp were connected to an EEG recorder. First she saw a flashing light, which produced one kind of brain-wave pattern. Then she heard a clicking sound, which produced quite a different pattern. When she was asked to count the flashes and clicks, instead of just watching and listening, her brain waves changed, producing new patterns. When she was asked to guess whether the next signal would be a flash or a click, her brain waves changed again. In fact, right guesses and wrong guesses left entirely different signatures in her brain-wave recording. Simply by reading her EEG records, Dr. Sutton was able to tell if the woman had been watching, listening, counting, or guessing, and if she was about to make a right or wrong guess.

Interpreting the data of an EEG can be something like mind reading. Dr. Sutton once described the awe he felt at being able to hand an assistant an EEG record and hear

To a specialist, an EEG has great significance. Dr. Montague Ullman studies a brain-wave recording at Maimonides Medical Center.

Harold Friedman, Maimonides Medical Center

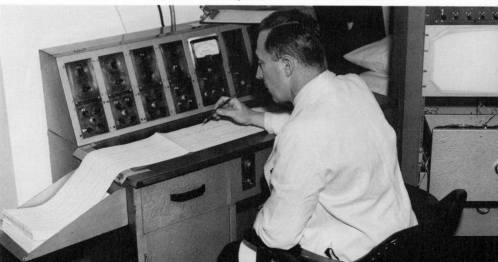

her say, "Oh, that's Jo Roberts when she makes a mistake," or, "That's Dorothy Jacobs when she knows ahead of time that she's going to see a flash of light." Not only was the assistant able to tell what had taken place by looking at the EEG's, but she was able to distinguish between the EEG's of Jo Roberts and Dorothy Jacobs.

No two people have exactly the same brain-wave patterns. The lines that appear on an EEG in response to a flashing light or a clicking sound will be roughly similar for most people, and yet each person's lines will be distinctive enough to serve as his brain's own personal signature. Even identical twins have different brain-wave patterns.

Brain waves can be detected in an infant, even before birth, but they are not organized like those of an adult. A newborn infant's brain waves appear on the EEG record as little more than a chaotic jumble of lines. Apparently, immature brain cells can produce nothing at first but meaningless baby talk. Before long, however, the squirming infant begins to gain some control over the movements of his body. As he does, his brain waves start to acquire definite rhythms.

Brain waves are usually classified by the frequency with which they occur—the number of electrical pulses per second. The waves most characteristic of the early months of life are slow *delta* rhythms, which occur with an average frequency of three electrical pulses per second. In healthy adults, these waves occur only during deep sleep. But in an adult whose brain has been damaged by injury or disease, slow delta waves may occur regularly.

As an infant grows older, the pace of electrical activity

in his brain quickens and other rhythms begin to take over. One of the typical rhythms of childhood are *theta* waves of about six pulses per second. These rhythms often are associated with emotions, both pleasant and unpleasant. They can be produced easily in a child by snatching away a toy he is playing with—or by giving him a new toy. However children, like adults, differ considerably in their brain-wave patterns. In some children theta waves are associated mainly with unpleasant feelings, in others mainly with pleasant ones. And in certain children, theta rhythms pop up regularly no matter what happens.

Until a child reaches the age of three or so, his EEG records could not possibly be mistaken for those of an adult. From three onward, however, the brain-wave rhythm typical of most adults begins to appear more and more often. This is the *alpha* rhythm which averages ten electrical pulses per second—about as fast as you can tap a finger. In some children, alpha rhythms may be fairly common by the age of four. However most children, until they are at least ten or eleven years old, show a mixture of ten-pulse-per-second alpha waves and six-pulse-per-second theta waves.

In adults, theta waves occur during light sleep and during daydreaming or reverie. Yet these rhythms may appear more often in adults who have highly emotional views about anything from politics to personal hygiene, or in unusually short-tempered or aggressive adults. Their impatience, selfishness and suspicion are mirrored in the juvenile appearance of their brain waves.

Momentary outbursts of theta activity can occur in any adult facing a disagreeable or frustrating situation.

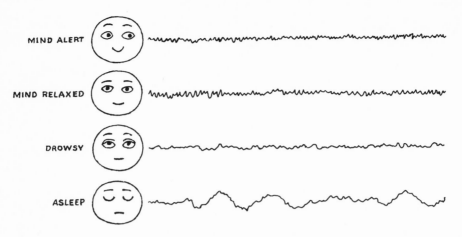

MIND ALERT

MIND RELAXED

DROWSY

ASLEEP

These typical brain-wave patterns reflect various states of mental alertness in a normal adult.

This happened once at a brain-wave laboratory in England, where a scientist had ordered a new machine for analyzing EEG's. The machine was delivered on a Saturday morning. By the time the scientist had adjusted it and was ready to try it out, several hours had passed. The only other person left in the lab was an off-duty technician who was listening to a championship soccer game on the radio. He agreed to help out as long as he could continue listening to the game.

The scientist pasted electrodes to the technician's scalp and began to test the new machine in the next room. Although he could not hear the radio, he soon realized that he could follow the progress of the game by watching the technician's EEG recording. When the recording began, the home team was leading and the technician's normal alpha rhythms droned on at about ten pulses per second, with only a trace of theta activity. But the game soon livened up and the visiting team pulled ahead. Every time the visiting team scored a goal, a sharp burst of theta activity appeared on the EEG graph.

As a rule, alpha waves provide the dominant rhythm of the relaxed but wakeful adult mind. Like searchlight beams swinging across the sky, these waves sweep regularly through the brain from front to back. They have been called "waves of inattention" because they are most prominent when the mind is not concentrating on anything in particular. During these periods, an individual's brain "idles" with a ten-pulse-per-second rhythm, producing a steady series of ripples on an EEG graph. But as soon as .the individual focuses his attention, his alpha waves tend to fade. A loud noise, a question, a disturbing thought, unexpected news—anything that distracts the mind from its inattention and causes it to focus—will flatten out the alpha waves and cause them to disappear momentarily from the EEG graph. Alpha waves are replaced in the alert mind by a faster, more irregular brain-wave rhythm with less amplitude, or strength.

In the laboratory, the standard way to interrupt the normal flow of alpha waves is to ask a person to do a simple arithmetic problem in his head. As he calculates, his alpha rhythms fade and his brain waves quicken. When he comes up with the answer, normal alpha activity begins again.

Ten-pulse-per-second alpha waves are most prominent when the mind is relaxed. When the mind is alerted, alpha waves are replaced by a faster brain-wave rhythm with less amplitude, or strength.

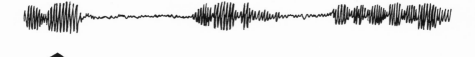

Scientists do not yet fully understand the significance of alpha rhythms. Since they tend to appear when the brain is not being bombarded with information, or is not involved in serious thought or problem solving, they may reflect a self-stabilizing process in the mind at rest. And yet alpha rhythms differ greatly from one person to another. These rhythms more than any others give each individual brain its own distinctive signature.

Without ever being aware of it, the average person slips in and out of alpha from five to thirty times a minute as his mind idles and then focuses. Among some people, however, alpha rhythms persist much of the time, even during concentration. Among others, these rhythms rarely occur at all. Instead, these people display an irregular brain-wave pattern with no fixed frequency.

Although alpha is the most prominent type of brain-wave activity, it seems to compete in the arena of the mind with faster-paced *beta* waves, which range from fourteen to thirty electrical pulses per second. Beta rhythms usually are associated with problem-solving situations, with intense concentration, and with tension and anxiety. In fact, the excited beta wave rather than the more relaxed alpha wave is typical of most people during any kind of hectic mental activity. Recent research has revealed that heavy smokers generate usually large amounts of beta activity and very little alpha activity.

At the State University of New York in Stony Brook, Dr. Lester G. Fehmi has found that gifted and creative people tend to spend more time than usual on alpha waves, even though they may be engaged in intensive work or study. Apparently, these people work best when their minds are relaxed. "There is a clear correlation between the presence of alpha waves and the absence of anxiety," says Dr. Fehmi. "It's the difference between 'psyching' yourself up for something and just letting things happen naturally."

Brain Waves and Personality

A famous authority on brain waves, Dr. W. Grey Walter of England's Burden Neurological Institute, has spent many years studying the relationships between brain waves, thinking, and personality. Dr. Walter believes that people can be divided into three major groups according to differences in their alpha-wave patterns.

One group consists of people who show hardly any alpha rhythms at all, even when their minds are completely relaxed. This is group "M" or "Minus," indicating the absence of significant alpha-wave activity. Dr. Walter has found that personality types designated as M think almost entirely in terms of colorful mental pictures. Mention the Fourth of July to an M-type and in his mind's eye he may see red, white, and blue flags, fireworks bursting in the air, holiday crowds on a bright summer day. When he thinks about his family, his job, his vacation, his income tax, or anything else, vivid Technicolor images are likely to flash through his mind.

A second group consists of people who have unusually persistent alpha rhythms which are not easily blocked out, even when their minds are actively involved. This is group "P" for "Persistent." Instead of forming mental pictures, people in this group think mainly in terms of words or abstract ideas. They also specialize in recalling sounds, movements, and the way things feel. To a P-type, the Fourth of July may bring to mind thoughts of independence, freedom, and equal rights for all. He may consider America's successes and failures at home, and her role as a world power abroad, but he is not likely to "see" vivid images. His mind's eye is almost blind. There seem to be about as many P-type individuals as M-types. Together they make up perhaps one-third of the population.

The remaining two-thirds of the population occupy a middle ground. They are called "R" types because they have "Responsive" alpha rhythms which appear when their minds are relaxed and disappear when their minds are alert. People in this group are likely to combine mental pictures, abstract ideas, and a variety of other impressions in their thinking. They can form visual images when they have to, but they usually will "see" only what is necessary. Though R-types tend to be more versatile and adaptable thinkers, they cannot visualize problems as readily as M-types, and they may not have the theoretical powers of P-types.

The most interesting thing about these groups is that they seem to reflect not only different ways of thinking, but also different personality types. Studies by Dr. Walter and his associates indicate that picture-thinking M-types and idea-oriented P-types tend to have clashing personalities and often find it difficult to get along with each other. Their different ways of thinking may lead to misunderstandings and even arguments they are unable to settle. Sometimes all it takes is a casual meeting and a brief exchange of words to make P- and M-types part company with ruffled feelings.

A personal experience of Dr. Walter's illustrates the possible clash between P- and M-types. He is known as a friendly, outgoing person who usually gets along well with his co-workers. A few years ago, however, he developed an intense aversion to a fellow researcher in his laboratory. As it turned out, the feeling was mutual, though neither man could offer a good reason for his dislike of the other. Later, when the lab began its study of personality types, it was discovered that Dr. Walter and the other scientist were opposite alpha-wave types. Dr. Walter was an extreme M-type, while his associate was a P-type.

Dr. Walter believes that clashes between different types might be avoided if these people were more aware that others do not always think exactly as they do. Actually, different ways of thinking can be complementary. Each person may have something important to offer in his way of looking at things. Taking these differences into account can spare feelings and at the same time help broaden a person's views.

Knowing an individual's brain-wave type could be an advantage in many areas of life. Schools, for example, might benefit from knowing the brain-wave types of their students. Certainly a child who finds it difficult to think visually should not be taught in quite the same way as one who easily forms mental pictures. In a survey called *The Making of a Scientist,* Ann Rowe found that picture-thinkers often have strong experimental inclinations. They can "see" what they want in an instrument or design and can start building with this picture in mind. Idea-oriented thinkers, on the other hand, often prefer theoretical work in science. They tend to analyze the evidence that supports certain findings, or the probability that a certain event will produce a certain result.

Information about an individual's thought patterns would certainly help teachers and counselors to guide students in the selection of an occupation. Someday, EEG tests may become standard tools to supplement traditional IQ, aptitude, and personality tests.

Knowledge of a person's alpha-wave type could also be useful in other ways. EEG tests might help select people who have to work or live in close quarters, such as members of submarine crews or space flights. Political leaders and diplomats might benefit too from having their EEG's typed. Can you imagine an international crisis developing because diplomats assigned to negotiate a disagreement were mis-matched alpha types and simply couldn't get along?

PROJECT

Testing Personality Types

Since the personality types described in this chapter are based on brain-wave patterns, it would be necessary to look at an EEG recording to determine accurately whether a person is a picture-thinking M-type or an idea-oriented P-type. However, Dr. W. Gray Walter has devised a simple test which may give some indication of the personality type to which an individual belongs.

Ask the person you are testing to shut his eyes and think of a painted wooden cube, like a child's block. Then ask him to imagine that he cuts this cube in half, from the top down. Now ask him to slice the cube again from the top down, making his second cut at right angles to the first one. When he has mentally made the first two cuts, have him make a third cut starting at the side of the cube and slicing it through the middle. Now ask your subject the following questions and record his responses:

1. Think of all the small cubes you have made. How many of their sides are unpainted? (You will find the answer with the project drawing; however, the important thing is how your subject arrives at his answer.)

2. Did you see the cube being cut?

3. What color was the cube?

4. Did you try to work out the answer mathematically, or did you visualize the little cubes in your mind?

People with different brain-wave types will usually have different answers to these questions. An M-type person, who produces few alpha waves, may say that the color of the cube was red or blue or yellow. He may also have seen the shine of the painted surface or the gleam of the saw blade as it cut through the block. He may even have seen sawdust falling as the block was cut.

A P-type person, one with persistent alpha waves, will probably say that no color was mentioned, or that the color doesn't matter. Yet this person may have heard the sound of the saw blade cutting the block and may have felt the roughness of the freshly cut sides. He may have arrived at his answer not by picturing the block as it was cut, but by

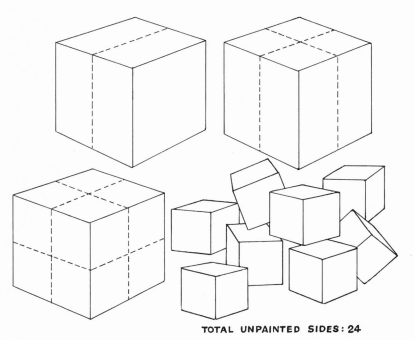

TOTAL UNPAINTED SIDES: 24

multiplying the final number of cubes by half the number
of their sides.

Individuals from the R group, those with responsive alpha
rhythms, may have pictured a block being cut. But they will
have seen only what was necessary for solving the problem
and may have combined what they saw with a little mathe-
matical calculation to arrive at their answer.

Test a large number of persons and record your results.
What percentage of your subjects seemed to be in each personality category? Do your results agree with those obtained
by Dr. Walter?

Tracking Down Signals from Sick Cells

In a hospital EEG lab, Dr. Donald Thomas adjusts the dials on a large brain-wave recorder, then signals his assistant to turn off the lights. The room is plunged into darkness. In one corner, an intense pink light begins to flash rapidly on and off. Like sheet lightning on a summer night, each flash illuminates the corner of the room for a split second, revealing a white pillow and the pale face of a patient lying quietly on a cot. Wire electrodes pasted to his scalp are plugged into the EEG machine that is recording his brain-wave activity.

After a few moments, the patient begins to complain of "strange feelings." The flickering light is making him feel faint and dizzy. Immediately, Dr. Thomas reaches for a switch, but before he can turn it off, the patient's arms and legs begin to jerk in rhythm with the flashing pink light. When the flashing light goes out, the patient quickly returns to normal.

The room lights are turned on again and the doctor begins to examine the EEG results. At the beginning of the test, wavy lines on the graph paper had depicted normal brain rhythms. Then these normal rhythms were interrupted by sudden deflections of the recording pens, producing sharply angled lines similar to those of a seismograph recording an earthquake. The trouble started in a small area of the brain, but as the EEG recording continued, the storm of electrical discharges seemed to sweep across large areas. This was a recording of an epileptic

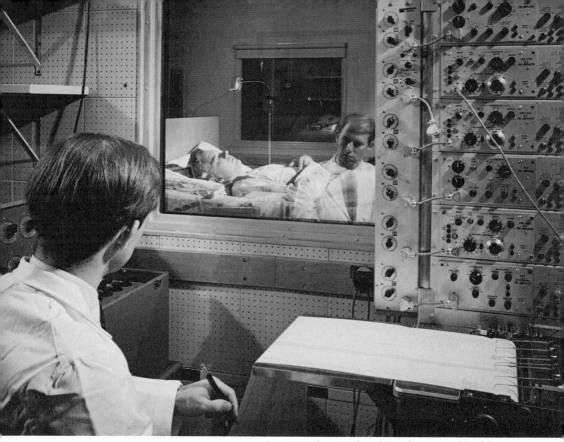

Brain-wave studies are used to diagnose epilepsy, tumors, and other brain disorders.

seizure—a mild "psychic fit" caused by the rhythmic flashes of the blinking pink light. Dr. Thomas had brought on the seizure intentionally to study the pattern of disturbances in the patient's brain waves.

People with epileptic tendencies seem to have certain super-sensitive brain cells. A flickering pink light can produce just the stress and tension necessary to make these cells start "firing" out of control. By triggering mild epileptic seizures in the laboratory, doctors can record what happens in the brain. Often they can locate the troubled area—the "sick cells" responsible for the seizure.

This is one of the first steps doctors take before deciding how to treat an epileptic patient.

Many other brain disorders also can be diagnosed with the aid of EEG records. Just as a fingerprint enables a criminologist to identify a suspect, a brainprint allows a doctor to do a little detective work. By studying a patient's brainprint, he may be able to track down damaged or diseased cells.

Ordinarily, EEG's are obtained by pasting electrodes to the scalp. But in cases of severe brain disorder, doctors will sometimes attempt to pinpoint the trouble by implanting electrodes deep inside a patient's brain. After a local anesthetic has deadened the nerves in the scalp, a tiny hole is drilled through the skull. As the patient's head is held firmly in position by the metal frame of a stereotaxic apparatus, thin wire electrodes are directed to a pre-determined site in the brain. The whole process is quite painless, and the patient feels no discomfort afterwards. The small wound in his scalp is closed over, but the electrodes are left in place so that they protrude slightly from miniature sockets cemented to the skull.

After the operation, the patient is free to follow his daily routine around the hospital ward. Several times during the day, and at night while he is sleeping, wires are attached to the electrode terminals that protrude from his head and EEG recordings are made. These records are analyzed and when the offending cells have been precisely located, doctors may decide to perform an operation in order to destroy or remove the trouble-making cells. Today there are thousands of people who have been helped by such operations.

Computers to the Rescue

In the early days of brain-wave research, scientists had great difficulty interpreting the brain's electrical language. One problem was caused by the vast amount of information that results from a single EEG recording session. In a routine twenty-minute session, more than half a million electrical pulsations from various parts of the brain may be recorded. This deluge of raw data tended to overwhelm early researchers. They had no efficient way of processing the information.

Another problem that confronted early researchers was background "noise." This confusing interference is caused by electrical activity in areas of the brain outside the specific area being studied. The pioneering brain-wave researcher was like a man trying to decode a message in a short-wave broadcast while interference and static drowned out the station to which he was tuned.

Today these problems are being overcome by sophisticated computers that can analyze brain-wave recordings almost instantly. Instead of spending hours of drudgery going over an EEG by hand, the researcher simply feeds raw data into the computer. It automatically screens out unwanted background noise and analyzes only the data the researcher wants to study. The computer accomplishes this by picking out brain-wave responses that occur again and again and by averaging those responses.

One computer intended especially for EEG research was designed by Dr. W. A. Clark, Jr., at the Massachusetts

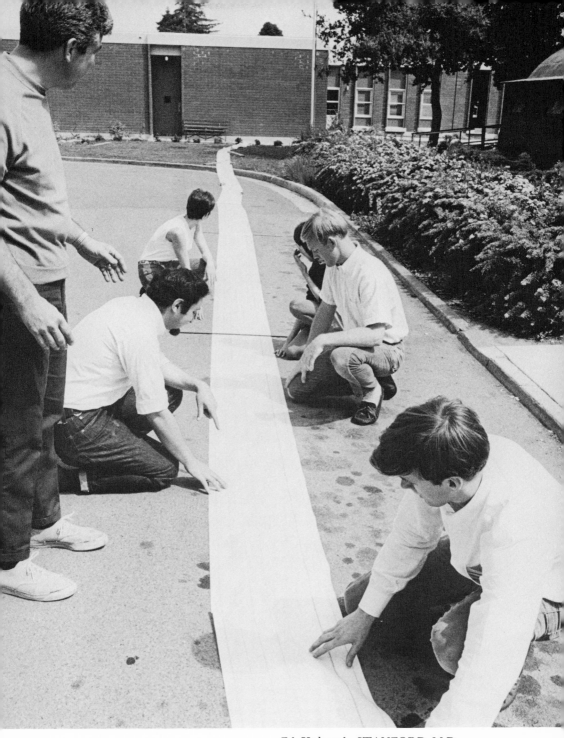

Ed Holcomb, STANFORD M.D.

An enormous amount of raw data may result from a single EEG
recording session. At the Stanford University Medical School,
researchers demonstrate the amount of work involved in analyzing
a brain-wave recording.

Institute of Technology. This high-speed electronic brain, called the Average Response Computer or ARC, processes brain-wave records as fast as raw data can be fed into it. At any time, the researcher can get an immediate feedback from magnetic tapes on which processed information is stored. This makes it possible to obtain average brain-wave results for a particular test even while the test is still going on.

With the aid of special-purpose computers, scientists are finding shades of meaning in the curves and angles of brain-wave recordings that were never dreamed possible a decade ago. At the Albert Einstein College of Medicine in New York, a computer has made it possible to identify the unique brain-wave pattern that represents the mental process of evaluation. If a person is trying to decide which of two things is more important, this pattern is always present. At Boston University Medical Center, scientists are using computers to measure the mind's attentiveness to a particular task. At UCLA, researchers believe that with computer-averaged EEG's it may soon be possible to know with certainty whether or not a person is telling the truth. And at New York Medical College, a new computer is analyzing the effects of drugs on brain-wave patterns. Scientists hope to find the characteristic signature of each drug's effects on the brain.

Hypnosis also is being investigated by EEG researchers using new computer techniques. The results are surpris-

(Right) Scientists at U.C.L.A. taught this chimpanzee to play ticktacktoe. As the chimp considers each move, his brain waves are analyzed by a computer. By determining whether or not the chimp is paying close attention, the computer can tell ahead of time if his next move will be right or wrong. The photo shows a mirror image of the hard-working chimp at play.

Leigh Wiener, U.C.L.A. Medical School

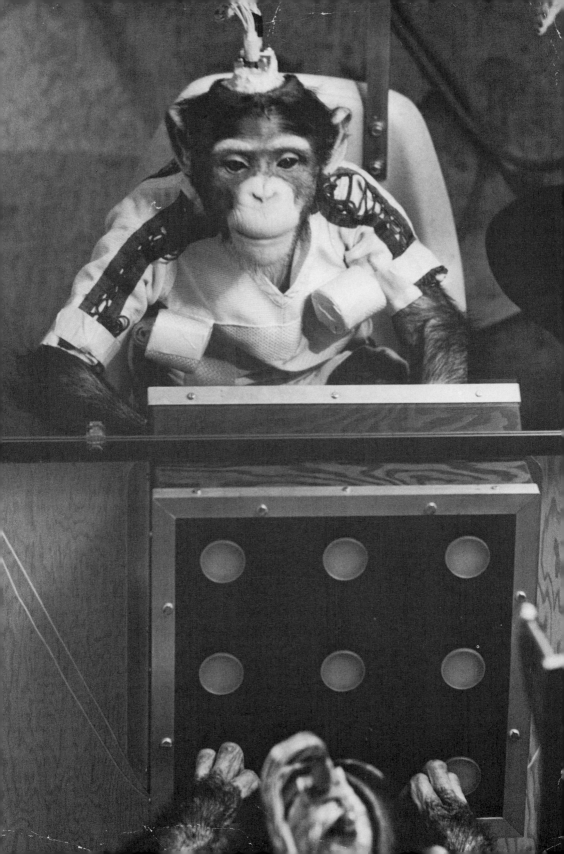

ing, since they indicate that a person under a hypnotic spell is not really in a state of sleep and that his brain responds normally to sights, sounds, and sensations. In other words, the EEG recordings do not reflect the hypnotist's influence on his subject. A hypnotized subject can be made to believe that a dim light is bright or a bright light is dim, but the "wool" is not pulled over the brain's eye. The subject's EEG responses reflect the actual brightness or dimness of the light, not the misleading suggestion made by the hypnotist. The subject can be convinced that he feels no pain when he is pricked with a sharp pin, and while he does not even flinch, his brain-wave patterns still say "ouch!" These studies indicate that the nature of hypnosis may be quite different from what it has appeared to be.

Advances in computer technology have unlocked a wealth of information never before available to EEG researchers. As a result, scientists are making dramatic progress in their continuing efforts to understand the electrical language of the brain.

CHAPTER *5*

Sleep and Dreams

The cat sat motionless, but her eyes darted back and forth as if following the movements of a mouse. Cautiously, she shifted into a crouching position. Her tail twitched and her whiskers quivered with excitement. Every muscle in her body seemed ready for the pounce.

Suddenly, with forelegs outstretched and claws extended, she leaped forward. But when she landed, there was only air between her paws. She had caught nothing. There was nothing for her to catch in the spotless, white-walled laboratory where she lived.

All the while, Dr. Michel Jouvet had been monitoring the electrical activity of the cat's brain. The wavy lines on the EEG graph indicated clearly that she was sound asleep.

Journey into Sleep

At research laboratories around the world, scientists are trying to find out what happens in the brains of animals and men when sleep closes the curtain of consciousness. In his own lab at the University of Lyon in France, Dr. Jouvet explained why the cat he was studying seemed to

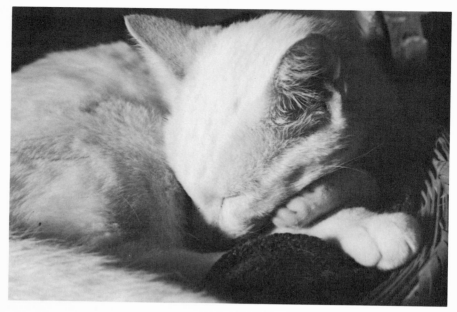

James E. Morriss

Sleeping cat. Is he dreaming?

be stalking a phantom mouse that had scampered through her dream.

Since most dreams occur when the body muscles are completely relaxed, dreamers do not usually get up and move around. However, Dr. Jouvet had been able to locate the small group of cells at the base of the brain that control muscular relaxation during dreaming. When he destroyed those cells, his experimental animals seemed to "act out" their dreams. They would get up, walk around, attack invisible enemies, and stalk imaginary prey. And all the time, their brain-wave recordings showed that they were sleeping.

Of course, we cannot be absolutely certain that the animals were dreaming, or even that animals dream at all. People can discuss their dreams at the breakfast table, but there is no way to "ask" an animal about its dreams. Yet indirect evidence, such as the sleep behavior of Dr.

Jouvet's cat, strongly indicates that many animals actually do dream.

Another experiment that suggests dream life in animals was performed with monkeys. They were trained to press a lever whenever certain pictures were flashed on a screen before them. After they had learned to do this, some of the monkeys were seen making lever-pressing motions in their sleep. Apparently, they were dreaming of the pictures they had been taught to respond to while they were awake.

Typical brain-wave rhythms associated with wakefulness in a cat (left), with light sleep (middle), and with deep sleep (right). Much of our current knowledge about sleep in both animals and humans has come from analyzing brain-wave recordings. *From "The States of Sleep," Michel Jouvet. Copyright © 1967 by Scientific American, Inc. All rights reserved.*

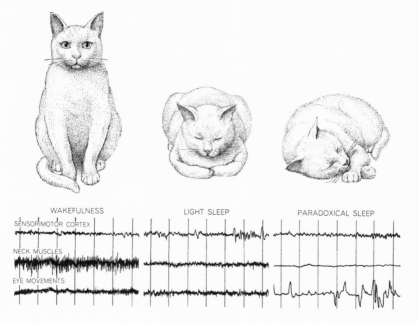

WAKEFULNESS   LIGHT SLEEP   PARADOXICAL SLEEP

SENSORIMOTOR CORTEX

NECK MUSCLES

EYE MOVEMENTS

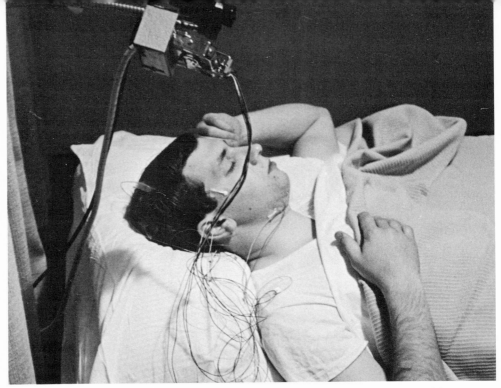

Jerry Hecht, National Institutes of Health

Wired for sleep: brain-waves, eye movements, breathing rate, and other physical functions are carefully monitored as a volunteer drifts into sleep.

Scientists have only recently started to unravel the mysteries of sleep and dreams. Much of what they have learned so far has come from analyzing brain-wave recordings taken during sleep. For the brain is never really at rest, not even during the deepest sleep.

A human spends perhaps a third of his life sleeping. And he spends twenty to twenty-five percent of each night's sleep dreaming. Human volunteers who participate in sleep studies get into bed each night with electrodes taped to their heads. The head is not the only part of the body that is wired. Temperature, blood pressure, breathing rate, eye movements, and muscle tone are all carefully recorded as the volunteer drifts into sleep.

These recordings provide clues to changes taking place in his body. And many changes do occur. One thing scientists have learned by comparing thousands of sleep recordings from volunteers is that one stage of a night's sleep may not be anything like another stage.

Each night when he goes to bed, a person passes through four distinct stages of sleep, each deeper than the one before. Stage one is the "drifting off" period, which may last only a few moments. Although the person is not fully asleep yet, consciousness becomes fuzzy and his brain waves begin to slow down.

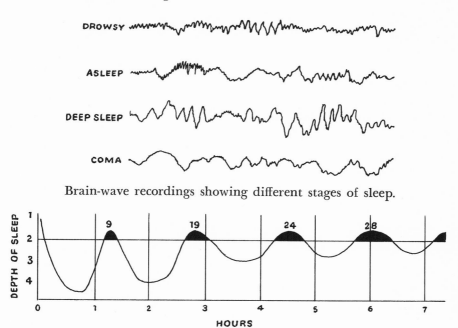

Brain-wave recordings showing different stages of sleep.

Sleep cycles: during the night a person sinks into deep sleep, rises toward lighter sleep, falls back into deep sleep, and so on. Rapid-eye-movements and dreaming begin each time the individual rises on the crest of lighter sleep. The length of each dream episode is shown by numbers at the top of the graph.

If he is not disturbed, the sleeper may then drift into stage two, or light sleep. He still can be awakened easily, but his EEG tracings indicate that a dramatic change has now occurred in his brain waves. Sharp bursts of electrical activity leave tight, jagged lines, called spindles, on the EEG graph. If he is awakened from this stage, the sleeper may insist that he wasn't really asleep at all.

As he sinks into stage three, slow rhythmical waves begin to appear among the spindles on the EEG graph. These are delta waves, ranging from one to three per second, and they indicate sound sleep. Blood pressure falls, breathing becomes regular and deep, and the muscles become more relaxed. A person is not easily awakened from stage three sleep.

About twenty to thirty minutes after the sleeper has first drifted off, the electroencephalograph begins to record slow delta waves exclusively. This is stage four, the deepest sleep of all.

Once he enters stage four, however, the sleeper does not remain there for long. After about ten to twenty minutes of deep sleep, he starts floating back up through the stages of lighter sleep toward consciousness. But he does not awaken. For the rest of the night he will ride the waves of the various sleep stages, rising toward lighter sleep, then falling into deep sleep. And each time he rises on the crest of lighter sleep, he will enter a strange new phase of his nighttime journey.

EEG recordings made during this phase of sleep look almost like those of alert wakefulness. Instead of the slow, regular delta rhythms of deep sleep, the brain-wave rhythms are fast and irregular. Breathing becomes un-

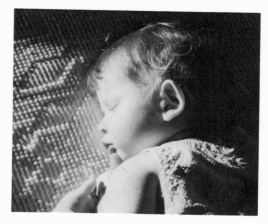

Barbara Secrest

Rapid-eye-movements behind slumbering lids indicate that infants dream more often than adults. What do they dream about?

even, and the heart rate and blood pressure shoot up. You would expect the person to be awakened easily, but this is not the case. Nothing short of a horn blast or calling his name loudly several times will rouse him. His muscles are completely relaxed. In fact, his body is totally limp. In some respects he seems to be fast asleep. In others, he seems nearly awake.

During this phase of sleep you can see the sleeper's eyes darting back and forth beneath his closed eye lids. Scientists refer to this phase as REM (Rapid Eye Movement) sleep. As the eyes move, it seems as if the sleeper is watching an action-packed movie in his sleep. Is he dreaming?

A person awakened from REM sleep will almost always report a dream. Even people who insist that they seldom dream, or who have difficulty remembering their dreams, will usually recall a dream-like experience when awakened from this phase of sleep. On the other hand, people awakened from non-REM sleep only rarely recall a dream. Recent research indicates that dreams may occur at any time during the night. But they seem to occur most often and most vividly when the sleeper is in that strange limbo between light sleep and deep sleep, when his muscles go limp, his heart pounds, his brain waves race, and his eyes jerk about behind slumbering lids.

The average person dreams four or five times each night, at regular intervals every eighty or ninety minutes. The first dream is usually a short one, lasting no more than five or ten minutes. When it is over, the sleeper may turn over in bed. Once again he sinks down into the depths of sleep, then drifts back up toward lighter sleep and another dream.

Early night dreams usually seem to be a jumbled re-hashing of events that have taken place during the day. As the night wears on, however, dreams become both longer and "dreamier." The last "late show" of the night may last from twenty-five to forty minutes and usually contains more unreal fantasies than earlier dreams.

Sleep cycles similar to those in man have been found in many of the higher animals, but not in all. Research in-dicates that coldblooded animals such as frogs and reptiles may never sleep. During their resting periods they are quiet and motionless, yet they are actually awake. Birds are warmblooded, and those birds that have been studied in the laboratory definitely do sleep. Chickens and

Sleeping hen. Chickens and other birds sleep deeply and undergo brief periods of REM or "dream sleep."

James E. Morriss

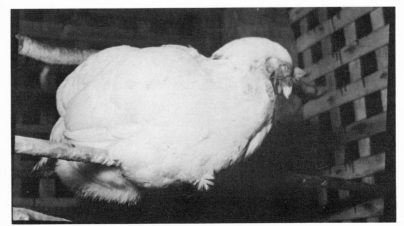

pigeons, for example, sink into a deep sleep characterized by slow brain-wave rhythms and go through brief periods of REM or "dream sleep." Both deep sleep and REM sleep also seem to occur in all mammals. However mammals differ greatly in their sleep habits.

Most mammals can be divided into two groups: "good sleepers" and "poor sleepers." The poor sleepers include vulnerable animals such as rabbits who are exposed constantly to danger. Sheep and goats, who doze in open pastures or on rocky mountain slopes where they may be attacked at any time, are also poor sleepers. These animals are usually nervous and excitable. They do not sleep as long or as deeply as the good sleepers and they spend very little time in REM or dream sleep.

Good sleepers include mammals such as ground squirrels and moles who slumber in the hidden security of a deep burrow. Moles sleep about eight hours a day, and like humans, spend about one-fourth of this time in apparent dream sleep. Chimpanzees, who spend their nights perched safely at the tops of trees, are also good sleepers. So are cats and other predatory animals who have few enemies. A grown cat spends about fourteen hours a day sleeping and seems to be dreaming twenty-seven percent of the time.

What do animals dream about? No one really knows. It is not uncommon to see a dog dozing in front of the fireplace as he jerks his legs back and forth and whimpers excitedly in his sleep. Is the dog chasing a dreamy rabbit? Possibly so. The famous psychologist Sigmund Freud believed that dreams are often wish fulfillments. "I do not myself know what animals dream of," he wrote. "But a proverb, to which my attention was drawn by one of my students, does claim to know. 'What,' asks the proverb, 'do geese dream of?' And it replies, 'They dream of grain.' The whole theory that dreams are wish fulfillments is contained in this proverb."

If dreams are wish fulfillments, then perhaps dogs really do dream of chasing rabbits, while cats dream of catching mice. Ground squirrels slumbering soundly in their hidden burrows may even dream of the perfect nut.

PROJECT

What's in a Dream?

One way to study dreams is to analyze their content. Two scientists, Calvin S. Hall and Robert L. Van de Castle, recently developed a method of analyzing dreams objectively. They placed the things people dream about into various categories, such as "Objects," "Settings," "Characters," etc. Then they kept score of the number of times these categories showed up in the dreams they studied. They found that what we dream about varies according to our age, sex, and life situation.

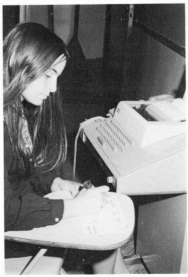

Joseph P. Cacossa

Lynn Orlowitz, a student at Division Avenue High School in Levittown, N.Y., uses the school computer to correlate the results of her own study of dream content with the results obtained in a similar study carried out by dream research scientists Calvin S. Hall and Robert Van de Castle. Lynn was selected to present her research at a recent Youth Science Congress, sponsored jointly by the National Science Teachers Association and the National Aeronautics and Space Administration.

Women dream in color more often than men, and the setting of their dreams is more often indoors or in a familiar place. Men's dreams, on the other hand, tend to be more adventurous and involve more physical activity. In women's dreams, male and female characters appear in about equal numbers, while in men's dreams male characters outnumber females two to one. Children dream of animals much more often than adults do—especially about unusual or frightening animals such as jungle creatures, bears, alligators, spiders, and insects. The four-year-olds studied had animal visitors in their dreams sixty-one percent of the time, while the adults had animal dreams only about eight percent of the time.

If you wish to make a study of dream content, you can begin by:

1. *Collecting dreams.* Ask members of your family and friends to keep a record of their dreams. Dreams are fragile things and are quickly forgotten once the day's activities begin, so a pad and pencil by the bed, or a tape recorder, will help your volunteer dreamers capture their dreams while the details are still fresh in their minds.

2. *Analyzing dream content.* Use the type of card shown on the next page to score the dreams you collect. Make out a separate card for each dream and count or check the items described in the dream. Organize the cards into groups you wish to compare. Possible groups might include: Male Adults, Female Adults, Male Children, Female Children, etc. For additional information on dream scoring you may wish to refer to *The Content Analysis of Dreams,* by Calvin S. Hall and Robert L. Van de Castle (Appleton-Century-Crofts, 1966). The sample card represents a simplified version of the scoring system used by Hall and Van de Castle.

DREAM SCORE CARD
Group: *Female Adult*

Name: *Betty Spector*
Dream No.: *12*

OBJECTS		SETTINGS		CHARACTERS		ACTIVITIES		EMOTIONS	
Buildings	/	Indoor		Male adults	/	Sitting	✓	Happiness	✓
Household	8	home	✓	Female adults	/	Lying		Sadness	
Food	3	school		Male children		Standing	✓	Confusion	
Money		work		Female children	/	Walking	✓	Anger	
Vehicles		away		Familiar	3	Running		Apprehension	
Tools	2	other		Strangers		Flying		Other	
Communication		Outdoor		Animals		Riding			
telephone		home		dogs		car			
radio-TV	/	etc.		cats	/	horse		COLORS	
other		Familiar	✓	spiders		other		Black & white	
Natural		Unfamiliar		monsters		Talking	✓	red	✓
trees		Day		other		Looking	✓	blue	
rocks		Night	✓	*hamster*	/	Thinking	✓	other	
other						Working		*yellow*	
Clothing	/					Fighting		*green*	
Other						Other			
						Eating	✓		

3. *Comparing dreams.* Be sure the total number of items scored is about the same for each group of dreamers you wish to compare. To obtain an accurate idea of which objects, settings, characters, etc., occur most often in the dreams of a particular group, you will need a large number of dream records. If this is not possible, you may wish to limit your study to the dreams of just a few individuals. Comparing the dreams of a child and an adult, or a boy and girl about the same age, may be just as interesting.

4. *Recording your results.* A bar graph such as the one shown below is ideal for recording your final results and comparing the content of the dreams you collect.

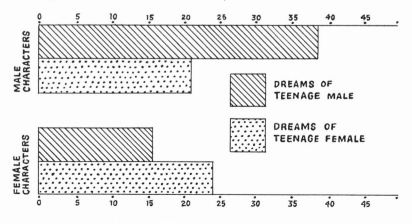

Why Do We Dream?

It is easy enough to see why a tired body needs a restful night's sleep. But what useful purpose might be served by the nighttime fantasies that dance through our sleeping brains? While scientists are not certain just what function dreams serve, experiments indicate that dreaming is important to humans and many animals as well.

At Stanford University, Dr. William Dement wondered what would happen if certain animals were allowed to get all the sleep they wanted but were prevented from dreaming. In one series of experiments, Dr. Dement deprived cats of their dream sleep. He did this by making each cat sleep on a brick surrounded by water. The cats had no trouble drifting into the early stages of sleep, since their muscle tone kept them from falling off the brick. Sitting on their little islands, they snoozed quietly until they finally reached the dream stage, or REM sleep. At this stage, muscle tone is lost completely and the body goes limp. Of course, Dr. Dement's cats never entered REM sleep, for as their bodies went limp they began to fall into the water.

A tom cat named Fyodor was deprived of REM sleep for seventy days. Fyodor had all the non-REM sleep he wanted. But his dream loss seemed to show. The old tom cat grew extremely restless and underwent definite personality changes. He became a real slob, neglecting to wash, and he was even caught dozing off in his litterbox.

Dr. Dement and his co-workers also have experimented

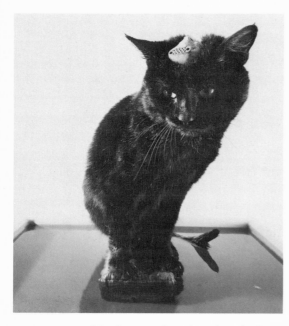

Crouched on a brick surrounded by water, a tomcat named Fyodor takes part in a dream deprivation experiment. For 70 days and nights, Fyodor was able to sleep but not to dream. Lack of dream sleep affected his behavior.

with dream deprivation in humans. In these experiments, volunteers were awakened every time their eye movements and brain-wave tracings indicated that they were slipping into REM sleep. With people, as with cats, the loss of dream sleep seems to show. After a while volunteers began to display anxiety. They became highly irritable and had difficulty concentrating. Those deprived of dreams for as long as fifteen days underwent temporary personality changes, becoming hostile and suspicious.

When dream deprivation ended, Dr. Dement observed a remarkable change in the sleep cycles of his volunteers. If a person is deprived of REM sleep on one night, his body will try to make up for the loss on the following night by increasing the amount of time spent dreaming. In fact, the body seems to have a built-in bookkeeping mechanism that keeps track of time spent in dream sleep. "How and why this happens," says Dr. Dement, "is the most fascinating biological puzzle of the decade." Since the body takes the trouble to make up for lost dream sleep, it would certainly seem that dreams must serve some important function in our lives.

There are a number of theories to explain what dreaming may do for us. Some psychologists believe that dreams act as a kind of safety valve. According to this view, dreams permit us to express thoughts and fulfill wishes that we ordinarily conceal from ourselves. During our waking hours we are not truly aware of these thoughts

At the Stanford University School of Medicine, Dr. William Dement tapes electrodes to the head of a volunteer in preparation for one of his experiments on sleep and dreaming.

Ed Holcomb, STANFORD M.D.

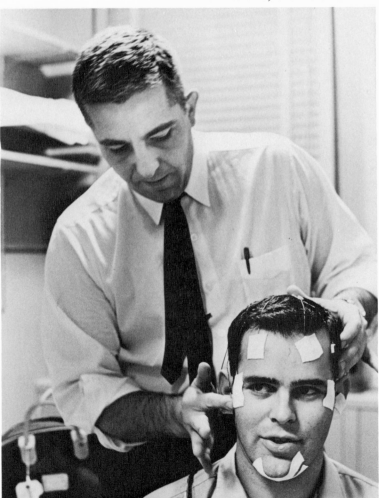

and wishes. We suppress them, as if hiding them away in some secret compartment of the mind. Even when these thoughts and wishes come out of hiding in our nighttime dreams, they often appear in disguise. For example, if a person wants to run away from a disagreeable situation, but can't admit this to himself, he may dream that he is taking a trip. The dream permits him to "act out" his forbidden wish as he sleeps.

Recent research has thrown new light on the mysterious world of our dreams. A number of scientists believe they now have good evidence to show that dreams play an important role in memory storage. "The results of many laboratory studies . . . during the past few years have led us to a completely new concept of the nature and function of sleep and dreaming," says Dr. Arthur Shapiro of the Downstate Medical Center in New York. According to Dr. Shapiro, the sleeping brain turns off most information coming from the outside world and concentrates on what has already been recorded.

"This housekeeping involves throwing out junk information and sorting out the specially important," he explains. "If useless information were allowed to accumulate, the storage capacity of the brain would be so clogged in a few days, it would no longer function properly. . . . The sorting and indexing of information that is not erased makes it easier for the brain to find it again. . . . If a happening during the day is significant, it must make a lasting impression. This can't be done on nerve tissue with just one occurrence. It has to be played over and over. This is where dreaming comes in. Some material taken in during the day is given low priority and dumped.

Other things are experienced over and over in dreams."

Do our dreams help us remember what is important? We know that the faces, voices and events of the day often turn up in our dreams. But how is it possible for the brain to file away a face, a voice or an event? How can the brain index a memory so that it can be called back into consciousness whenever we want to remember?

CHAPTER *6*

Memory and Intelligence

The ancient Greeks thought of the mind as a blank slate on which the fingers of experience "wrote," as a secretary writes down dictation in her notebook. When we try to remember a line from a poem or an old friend's name, we are in a sense searching through our minds' old notebooks. But what exactly are these notebooks? How does experience scribble its impressions on the living tissue of our brains?

Scientists agree that memories must leave some kind of trace in the brain. Otherwise they would be completely lost. The search for this memory trace has gone on for many years and continues to be one of the most fascinating fields of scientific investigation.

What Is Memory?

A few decades ago, Dr. Karl S. Lashley of Harvard University spent an enormous amount of research time trying to discover where specific memories are filed away in the brain. He taught laboratory rats to solve certain problems, such as finding their way through a maze in order

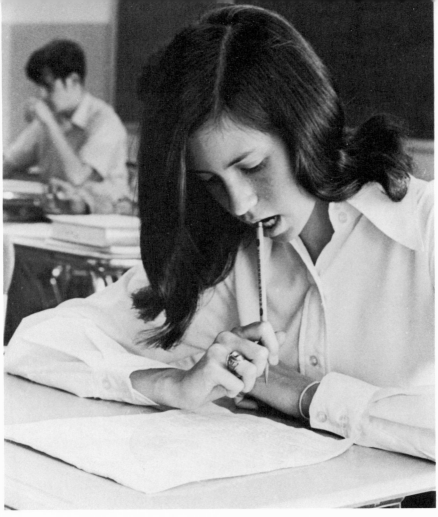

What happens in the brain when we try to remember?

to find food. After training the rats, he removed portions of their brains in hopes of locating those areas where the memories were stored. But no matter what part of the brain he removed, the rats were still able to remember and perform the tasks Dr. Lashley had taught them.

Even when huge portions of their brains were taken out, the rats remembered some part of what they had learned. Of course, the more brain tissue Lashley removed, the fuzzier the rats' memories seemed to become. If he removed twenty-five percent of the cerebral cortex —the outer covering of the brain—the rats were able to remember about seventy-five percent of the problem. If he removed fifty percent of the cortex, they remembered about half the problem.

These experiments seemed to indicate that memories are not laid down in any specific area of the brain, but are spread out over large areas of the cortex. Dr. Lashley's results certainly were puzzling. Memory seemed to be nowhere in particular and everywhere in general.

After years of painstaking research, Dr. Lashley had to confess that his investigations had "yielded a good bit of information about what and where memory is not." If memories are stored in any specific part of the brain, Lashley had not been able to uncover that storehouse.

During the 1950's, a startling new discovery seemed to contradict Dr. Lashley's findings. The discovery was made by Dr. Wilder Penfield, director of the Montreal Neurological Institute. A noted brain surgeon and researcher, Dr. Penfield was already well known for his work in mapping large areas of the cerebral cortex in the human brain. Using an electric probe to stimulate the cortex, he had been able to pinpoint certain areas that control muscular movement and other areas that receive messages from the senses. Now, while performing a brain operation on one of his patients, he had accidentally located what seemed to be a storehouse for certain memories.

This brain operation, like many others, was being performed with a local anesthetic which deadened only the nerves in the scalp, where a small section of skin and bone had been removed to expose the brain. The patient remained conscious, sitting upright in a chair. As Dr. Penfield probed the delicate tissue of the cortex in search of damaged brain cells, the patient was able to speak and could describe her thoughts and feelings.

Suddenly she recalled a song she had once heard and had long since "forgotten." The memory was so vivid, it was like listening to a phonograph. And the "phonograph" in the patient's head could be turned on and off with Dr. Penfield's electric probe. When the probe was removed, the song stopped. When the same area was stimulated again, the song started.

When Dr. Penfield stimulated another area of the cortex, the patient remembered a childhood experience. This scene from the past appeared so clearly and in such

A patient receiving electrical stimulation of the brain is questioned by a psychiatrist at Massachusetts General Hospital. In the foreground, a physician records the patient's brain-wave reactions.

John Loengard, LIFE *Magazine* © *Time Inc.*

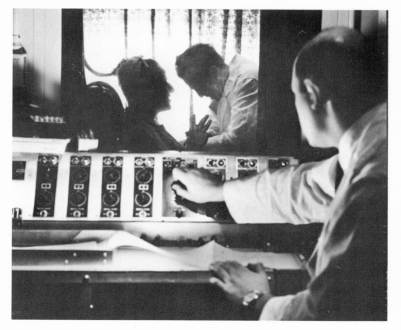

minute detail, the patient was able to remember colors, sounds, and smells, and was able to recall exactly how she had felt at the time. It was like living through the experience all over again.

As he performed similar operations on other patients, Dr. Penfield was able to tap a variety of memories that the patients had not recalled for many years. In each case, his electric probe brought back those memories with incredible accuracy and realism. It certainly seemed that the Canadian physician had pinpointed specific memory sites in the brain.

Before long, however, the memory mystery deepened again. Dr. Penfield's own co-workers found that if a specific memory site was removed from a patient's brain during an operation, those memories were *not* lost after all. The patient was still able to remember the experience he had recalled before the operation. Evidently, other parts of the brain were involved in the total memory experience. As Dr. Lashley had found in his earlier experiments with rats, specific memories seemed to be spread throughout the cerebral cortex.

As scientists tried to discover *where* the brain stores its memories, they also attempted to learn exactly *how* memories are filed away. One widely held theory suggested that electricity was the key to memory storage. According to this view, electrical impulses entering the brain caused permanent changes of some kind in the connections between brain cells. Many scientists suspected that memories were actually faint electrical echoes, reverberating endlessly through nerve pathways in the brain.

When we recall a memory, are we tuning in on these electrical echoes? If so, then it should be possible to destroy memory by erasing the electrical activity of the brain.

This approach was tried by a number of scientists experimenting with laboratory animals. They tested various methods of destroying the electrical echoes that were suspected to be the basis of memory. Animals were given powerful drugs. Their brains were frozen, heated, and subjected to severe shock. All of these methods disrupted or shut down the brain's electrical activity and should have destroyed electrically based memories. But this did not happen. When the animals recovered, they still remembered skills they had learned. At least, they remembered sometimes. For scientists now discovered that there is more than one kind of memory.

If a rat is taught a new trick, and is immediately given an electric shock to short-circuit the electrical activity of his brain, he will forget what he has learned. If half an hour passes before the shock is given, he will remember part of what he has learned. However, his memory may be faulty or blurred, like a negative that is exposed to light before it is completely developed. If several hours pass before the shock is given, the rat will remember everything he has learned. The memory has apparently been "fixed" in his brain.

These experiments indicated that there are two kinds of memory: short-term memory and long-term memory. Short-term memory is the kind we use to remember a telephone number just long enough to dial it. Scientists believe that these memories are probably electrical in nature

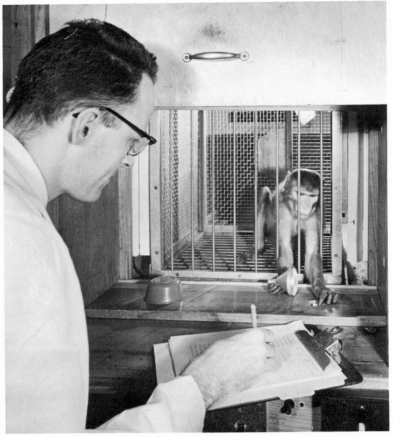

Where's the peanut? In this memory test, the monkey must remember which cup he lifted last in order to lift the correct one on his next trial. Between trials, the cups are hidden by a screen for periods ranging from a few seconds to many minutes. The monkey is rewarded with a peanut if he remembers to lift the cups in a simple alternating sequence: left, right, left, and so on.

and that they disappear quickly unless they are converted into more permanent long-term memories.

Recent experiments suggest that long-term memories may be stored *chemically* in the brain. According to a new theory, these memories are recorded in tiny chemical packages called molecules, which are filed away in the brain like pictures in an album.

Search for the Memory Molecule

The first real breakthrough in the search for the brain's memory mechanism took place not long ago in the laboratory of Dr. Holger Hydén at the University of Göteborg in Sweden. Dr. Hydén knew that the rich electrical activity of the brain is paralleled by an equally rich chemical activity. Brain cells are living generators and transmitters of electricity, but they are also remarkably active chemical factories. In fact, brain cells exceed all other body cells in their ability to manufacture proteins, a special group of chemical substances found in all living matter.

One kind of protein manufactured in large quantities by brain cells is *ribonucleic acid,* or RNA. This substance is so plentiful that 20 million or more RNA molecules are found in every one of the brain's nerve cells. RNA molecules act as chemical "foremen." They direct the manufacture of other kinds of protein molecules the cell needs to grow and function properly.

Working in his laboratory in Sweden, Dr. Hydén found that the amount of RNA in the brain increases as a young animal grows up and acquires new experiences. This increase seems to be caused by stimulation of the senses. The more information the animal picks up from its surroundings, the more RNA is manufactured by its brain cells. On the other hand, if the animal is deprived of one of its senses, such as hearing, the brain cells that normally receive stimulation from that sense will not develop as they should. These cells are like empty bags, impoverished in both RNA and other molecules.

Since the RNA content of brain cells depends on the amount of stimulation those cells receive through the senses, it seemed possible that RNA molecules might be the "blank slate" on which the finger of experience writes. Dr. Hydén suspected that RNA might actually be the stuff memory is made of.

Hoping to discover more about the relationship between RNA and memory, the Swedish scientist decided to analyze the chemical content of brain cells before and after learning had occurred. This meant that individual cells smaller than a grain of dust had to be placed under a microscope and taken apart so they could be chemically analyzed. Dr. Hydén spent years developing a technique for removing single cells from the brain and then analyzing them. After isolating a cell, he would cut it open with a micro-scalpel. Then he would scrape out its contents so he could measure the amount and kind of RNA present.

After isolating a single brain cell, Dr. Holger Hydén would cut it open and scrape out its contents with a micro-scalpel. This photo illustrates the delicate technique developed by the Swedish scientist.

James E. Morriss

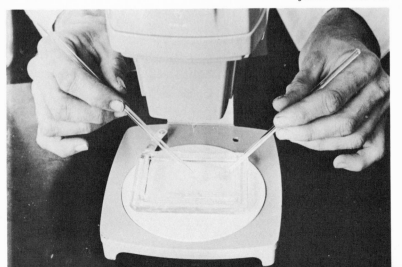

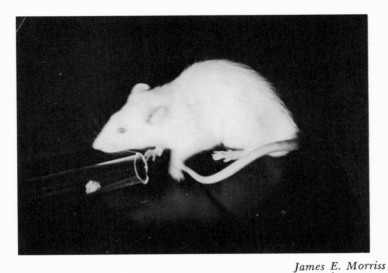

A left-handed rat, trained to use its right paw to get food from a tube, produces a special kind of RNA.

The cells Dr. Hydén studied were taken from rats, rabbits, and other animals he had trained in his laboratory. He found that any kind of training or experience increased the amount of RNA in the cells he studied. But he also discovered that different kinds of experience produced different kinds of RNA. In one experiment, Dr. Hydén trained rats to balance on a tightwire. Other rats were given an equal amount of exercise but did not learn anything new. Brain cells from animals in both groups showed a significant increase in RNA content. However, the RNA taken from rats that had learned to walk the tightwire was chemically different from the RNA of the untrained rats. Was this difference due to the difference in what the rats had experienced? Had the learning experience of the trained rats somehow been encoded in the RNA molecule itself?

Similar results were obtained in experiments at other laboratories. A lefthanded rat, taught to use its right paw to get food out of a tube, produced a special kind of RNA. Goldfish taught to swim with buoyant plastic foam under their chins produced another kind of RNA. Some researchers were even able to detect differences between samples of RNA taken from animals during early and late stages of learning. Had these scientists caught memory in the act of being formed?

Since RNA's job in the cell is to control the production of other protein molecules, Dr. Hydén believes that memories may be "printed" into these new molecules. In this way, dozens of copies of a memory could be produced and distributed throughout the brain. This would explain why earlier researchers were unable to destroy memory by removing certain sections of the brain.

Dr. Hydén's research has sparked a growing interest in the biochemistry of learning and memory. Dozens of other scientists all over the world have undertaken similar experiments with a wide variety of animals. From the evidence accumulated so far, it seems that RNA, if not the memory molecule itself, is at least an important link in the complicated chain of electro-chemical events that produces our remembrance of things past.

One of the many scientists impressed with Dr. Hydén's findings was James McConnell, a University of Michigan psychologist whose laboratory is awash with worms. Dr. McConnell chose flatworms, or planarians, to use in his investigations of memory because they may be the most primitive animals capable of learning. Worms are the simplest form of life to have a brain.

Planarians live at the bottoms of ponds and in rivers and streams. Like many other lower forms of life, they have the remarkable ability to regenerate. If a worm is cut into two or more pieces, each piece will grow into a complete new worm. Dr. McConnell wondered what would happen if he trained a worm and then cut it into two parts—a head half and a tail half. When the two halves regenerated, would they both remember what the original worm had learned?

Worms can be taught a variety of simple lessons. They can learn to swim through mazes, to crawl along a white

Educated worm: Dr. James McConnell trains a planarian to swim through a simple T-maze.

Planarian Research Group, University of Michigan

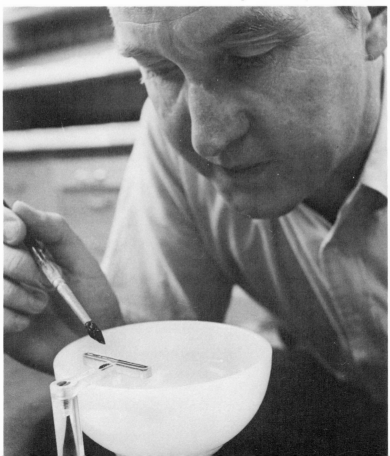

line, and to curl up at the signal of a flashing light. McConnell trained his worms to respond to a light. When the training was completed, these educated worms were cut in half. During a four-week layoff, their heads regenerated new tails and the tails grew new heads. Then all the new worms were tested for their ability to remember the lesson they had learned. Dr. McConnell was astounded to find that the original tails remembered almost as well as the original heads.

These results were hard to believe at first. Yet the experiment was repeated several times with the same result. The "heads or tails" test seemed to demonstrate that while learning takes place in the brain, memory of what is learned may be retained throughout the body. Even when worms were cut into three or four pieces, each of the regenerated worms retained some memory. Were the memories being duplicated in some kind of chemical code and distributed throughout the body?

At this point, McConnell wondered if it would be possible to transfer memory from the body of one planarian to the body of another. To begin with, he tried without success to graft pieces of trained-worm bodies onto the bodies of untrained worms. Finally he settled on a much simpler method. Since planarians thrive on almost any kind of food, including a diet of their fellow worms, McConnell decided to chop up some trained worms who had learned to curl up at a flashing light and feed them to untrained worms.

Would the untrained worms benefit from their "educated" diet? They certainly seemed to. From the very beginning, worms fed an educated diet learned to curl up at a flashing light faster than worms fed an uneducated diet. The fast learners had apparently taken in the memory of the flashing light along with their meals of fellow flatworms.

PROJECT

Will Tails Remember What Heads have Learned?

When a planarian is exposed to bright light, it will normally lift its head, stretch its body full length, and swim or crawl away. When it is disturbed by a sudden jarring vibration, the opposite reaction will occur. It will stop crawling and curl up. If a bright light is turned on and is immediately followed by a jarring vibration, the planarian will learn that the light is a signal which tells it that a vibration is coming. Once a planarian has learned to associate the light with the vibration, it will start to curl up as soon as the light goes on. This new response to light is called a *conditioned response,* since curling up (the response) was not originally caused by the light (the condition).

You can obtain planarians and information on their care and feeding from any biological supply house. A common fresh-water species which is widely distributed throughout the United States is *Dugesia tigrina.* Many investigators prefer this species for conditioning experiments. For further information about planarians, and a detailed description of experiments in conditioning and transfer of learning, we suggest you obtain *A Manual of Psychological Experimentation on Planarians.* A copy may be purchased by writing to Box 644, Ann Arbor, Michigan 48107.

1. A small, shallow plastic dish, such as a butter dish, can be used as a conditioning trough in which to train your planarians. The dish should be light in color so that the worms' responses can be seen easily. Be sure the dish is thoroughly cleaned and rinsed the first time it is used. Fill it with about a half-inch of spring water (bottled spring water can be obtained in any supermarket). Scientists who have trained planarians have found that they obtain better results when the water is changed at the beginning of each daily training session. Leave the same water in the dish between sessions.

2. Fasten the dish as tightly as possible to a piece of hardwood with a thick rubber band or heavy cord. Attach a loud buzzer or doorbell to the wood alongside the dish, and connect the buzzer or bell to a six volt battery. A push-button switch will allow you to turn the buzzer on and off with ease. Test the buzzer you intend to use to make sure it produces enough vibration to make your worms curl up.

3. The light source should be from a 75 to 150 watt bulb, housed in a ten-inch reflector and mounted about six to eight inches above the top of the conditioning trough. When you are training your worms, you must turn on the light *just before* you set off the jarring vibrations with the buzzer or bell.

4. Keep a record of your daily training sessions and record the responses your planarians make during each trial. Make from twenty-five to fifty trials a day with rest periods between each trial so the worms do not tire. It may take 150 trials or more before the worms learn their lesson.

5. How many trials were necessary before your worms responded by curling up as soon as the light was turned on?

6. Were fewer trials necessary to produce the same response on the following day?

7. After your worms have learned, wait a few days and then test them again. Did the worms remember what they had learned?

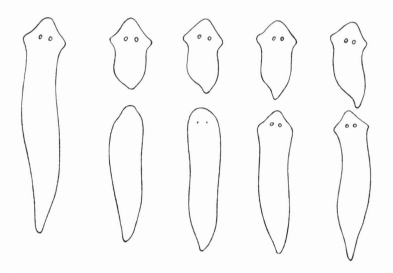

8. Once your worms are conditioned to curl up at a light, place them on a smooth block of softwood and cut them in half with a clean sharp razor. Allow the head and tail ends to regenerate in separate containers. After the heads have grown new tails and the tails have grown new heads, test the planarians again. How many trials are necessary before the head ends curl up as soon as the light goes on? How many trials are necessary for the tail ends? Do both halves relearn the response to light more quickly than the original untrained worms?

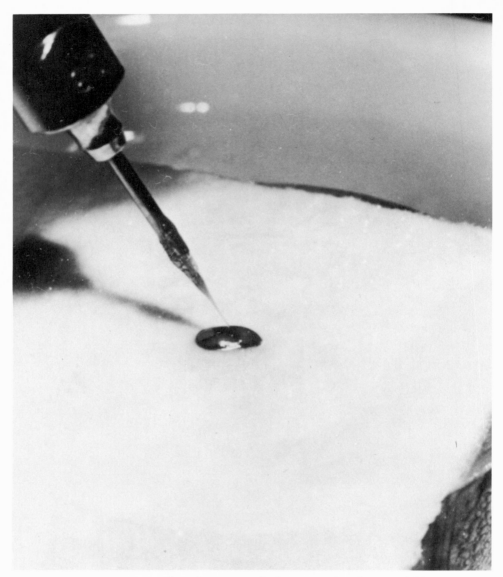

Planarian Research Group, University of Michigan
Learning by injection: a planarian being injected with RNA.

If memory can be transferred between primitive planarians, can it be transferred in higher forms of life? At
first, many scientists were skeptical. In fact, some scientists
still found it difficult to believe that memory could be

transferred at all. Yet it wasn't long before other researchers moved up the ladder from worms to mammals in their attempts to transfer memories from one animal to another.

At the University of California at Los Angeles, Dr. Allan L. Jacobson conducted transfer-of-training experiments with rats and hamsters, injecting brain matter from trained animals into untrained animals. He succeeded not only in transferring training from rats to rats, and from hamsters to hamsters, but also from hamsters to rats.

Many other scientists now began transfer-of-training experiments. At first, not all of them succeeded in getting the successful results reported by Jacobson and McConnell. At one point, twenty-two scientists from nine different research centers signed a report stating that they had tried to duplicate the results of Jacobson's experiments and in every case had failed. But two months later, a leading signer of the report, Dr. William L. Byrne of Duke University, changed his mind when he finally obtained successful results in an experiment. "Memory transfer is a real phenomenon," said Byrne. Others also began to change their minds as more and more experiments seemed to provide evidence that certain kinds of learning can indeed be acquired by untrained animals through injections of brain extract from trained animals.

At Baylor University College of Medicine in Texas, Dr. Georges Ungar tried a memory transfer experiment with mice. He placed one group of mice in a small cage and subjected them to a loud, clanging noise. At first the mice crouched and quivered in fear. But after a while they learned that the noise signaled no harm and

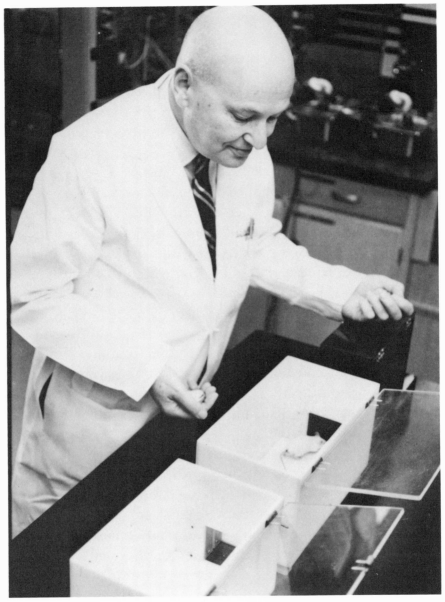

Baylor College of Medicine

Dr. Georges Ungar watches a mouse hesitate at the entrance to a dark box. Although mice normally prefer darkness, this mouse will not enter the box because it has been injected with scotophobin, a chemical that causes fear of darkness in both mice and rats.

they went about their business as usual. Once the mice had learned to ignore the noise altogether, Dr. Ungar sacrificed them, minced up their brains, and injected this educated brain broth into untrained mice. The first time the untrained mice were subjected to the clanging noise, they ignored it. They had apparently received an education by injection.

Dr. Ungar next experimented with rats, which normally avoid lighted places. They prefer the dark. The scientist set up a darkened box and a brightly lighted box and connected them with a narrow tunnel. Then he placed his rats in the lighted box. Every time they tried to scurry through the tunnel into the darkened box, they were jolted by an electric shock. The rats soon changed their natural preference. They learned to live in the light and to fear darkness. By preparing injections of brain broth from these trained animals, Dr. Ungar was able to transfer their fear of darkness to untrained rats.

Recently, Dr. Ungar reported success in isolating the chemical substance which, he believes, contains the fear-of-darkness memory. He also has produced an artificial or synthetic substance that is similar enough to produce the same fear when injected into untrained animals. Dr. Ungar calls this substance *scotophobin,* which means "fear of darkness."

If scientists can actually synthesize "memory molecules" in a test tube and inject them into an animal's brain, how soon will they be able to do the same for man? Would scotophobin produce fear of darkness in humans as well as rats? What other memory molecules will scientists be able to identify and produce artificially in the laboratory?

Will it someday be possible to get injections of courage or musical talent, algebra or French?

Memory Pills and Super IQ's

It may be a long while, if ever, before we can get our education by injection or buy bottles of musical ability and higher math. But there are available today an ever-increasing number of drugs that enhance memory and learning, and even a few that wipe out memories altogether.

At the University of Michigan Medical School, Dr. Bernard W. Agranoff trained goldfish to avoid an electric shock by swimming across a barrier in their tank. Most goldfish learn this task easily and remember it for many days. However, if a drug called puromycin is injected into the fish a few seconds after their learning trials, they will not remember their shock-avoidance lessons. On the other hand, if an hour is allowed to pass before the drug is injected, their memories are not affected. Apparently, this drug is able to erase a memory before it becomes permanently fixed in the brain.

Other drugs that interfere with memory are now being tested. Soon there may be a wide variety of chemical compounds which will, when injected or swallowed in tablet form, destroy memories altogether.

Many drugs that seem to improve memory and learning ability are also being tested today. One memory drug, magnesium pemoline, seems to enhance the production of RNA in the brain. When this drug was tested on rats, scientists found that it increased their learning ability

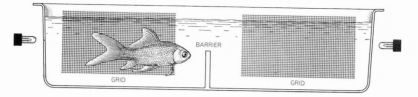

Training tank for goldfish: after the fish learned to swim over the barrier, their memories were erased. *From "Memory and Protein Synthesis," B. W. Agranoff. Copyright © 1967 by Scientific American, Inc. All rights reserved.*

significantly. And its effects on learning seemed to last. Later, the same drug was tested on humans. At the Veterans Administration Hospital in Albany, New York, Dr. D. Ewen Cameron gave magnesium pemoline to patients who had suffered severe memory losses. Some of the patients recovered sufficiently to leave the hospital and return to work. The drug was also effective in improving the memories of elderly patients who were suffering from senility. One man had forgotten how to turn on a TV set. Another, who had once been a good bridge player, had forgotten the game. With magnesium pemoline, the memories of these patients improved and they were able to lead more normal lives.

Another drug, ribaminol, has been tested on animals, on elderly hospital patients, and on university students. Ribaminol affects the production of brain protein, and in some cases it produced a twofold increase in learning ability. Its effects seemed to last for several months after the animal or human subjects had stopped receiving the drug.

At the University of California in Riverside, Dr. James L. McGaugh and his co-workers have been investigating the effects of a drug called metrazol, which stimulates the central nervous system and helps convert short-term re-call into long-term memory. Dr. McGaugh tested this drug on two groups of mice with different hereditary backgrounds. Mice in one group were a good deal smarter than those in the other group. When all the mice were given a certain amount of metrazol, they showed a forty percent improvement in learning ability over mice that did not receive this drug. If metrazol was given only to the genetically backward mice, they performed at least as well as the brainier mice. In fact, after injections of metrazol, some of the "stupid" mice became better learners than their genetically brighter cousins.

How will society use the new galaxy of mind-affecting drugs?

Parke-Davis

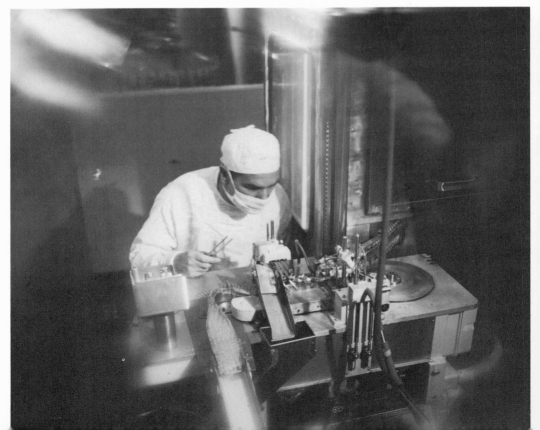

As yet, no one really knows how effective and useful these experimental drugs will prove to be. If the new "smart pills" and memory drugs do nothing but restore the learning capacity of older people to that of their younger years, they can provide a valuable service. And yet the potential use and abuse of drugs that can raise the level of intelligence as well as wipe out memory raises frightening social questions. One danger is that these drugs could be administered to people without their knowledge. Another is that, in a controlled society, mind-improving drugs might be given to some people and withheld from others. Man has been developing his brain for a million years or more, and now, within the past few years, he has suddenly discovered the means to intervene in that development.

Speaking before a sub-committee of the U.S. Senate, Dr. David Krech of the University of California warned that the day is fast approaching when society will have to decide how the new galaxy of mind-affecting drugs will be used. "Brain research," he said, "is immeasurably more significant for the future of man than anything now going on in science. . . . I foresee the time when we shall have the means, and therefore the temptation, to manipulate the behavior and intellectual functioning of all people. . . . If we fail to prepare ourselves for that eventuality, then we might find it too late to institute effective, carefully thought through, and humane controls."

Along with many other scientists and concerned citizens, Dr. Krech believes that the time for society to consider the consequences of modern brain research is now.

CHAPTER *7*

Behavior by Remote Control

The "boss monkey" was in a nasty mood. This powerful old male was the leader of Yale University's monkey colony and he ruled his subordinates with an iron hand. Just now his anger was being directed at a small, frightened male with downcast eyes who had stepped out of line. It appeared that the little monkey was in for trouble.

The old boss shook his head furiously and began to scream at the young male. Suddenly, the little monkey rushed over to one side of the cage, reached through the bars, grabbed a switch on an instrument panel, and with a quick jerk pulled the switch. Then he wheeled around and did something that is absolutely forbidden in monkey society. He stared his boss right in the eye.

A rhesus monkey never looks directly at a superior, especially if that superior happens to be the boss monkey himself. Ordinarily, the boss would not put up with such insolent behavior. But this was no ordinary situation. As the little monkey stared defiantly at him, the boss turned quietly away. His rage of a moment before seemed to disappear. He was responding not to the disrespectful look of his inferior, but to a radio signal.

The monkeys were taking part in brain-stimulation experiments conducted by Dr. José Delgado and his associates at Yale. Strapped to the boss monkey's back was a small transistor radio receiver. It was connected to wire electrodes buried deep inside the boss's brain. When the little monkey pulled the switch outside the cage, radio waves picked up by the receiver were relayed to the boss's brain, blocking his aggressive drive and making him forget his anger.

Dr. Delgado has pioneered in developing new techniques of ESB—electrical stimulation of the brain. When

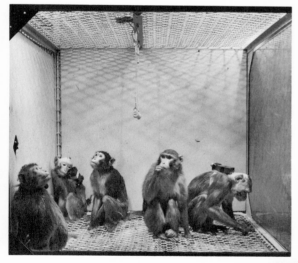

John Loengard, LIFE *Magazine* © *Time Inc.*

(Left) Monkeys at Yale sit peacefully in their cage. Note radio receivers strapped to their backs. The monkey at far right is about to be given ESB by remote radio command.

(Right) As radio signals are transmitted to his brain, the monkey goes into a fierce rage and terrorizes his companions.

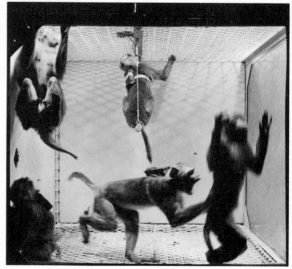

he first started his research, electrodes planted in the brain had to be connected to a power source by means of long wires. This method worked well enough with rats, cats, and other experimental animals, but monkeys often became curious about the trailing wires and pulled them out of their sockets. Dr. Delgado developed a monkey-proof method of ESB by replacing the plugged-in-wires with portable radio receivers. These receivers pick up signals broadcast by a distant transmitter and convert the signals into electrical impulses, which are then relayed to electrodes in the brain.

By remote radio command, Dr. Delgado has been able to control the behavior of a variety of animals. If radio signals are transmitted to the muscle-controlling area of an animal's brain, the animal will move various parts of its body. Like an electronic toy, it can be commanded to open or close its mouth, wink its eyes, turn its head, stand up, sit down, walk about, and turn around. If radio signals are transmitted to deeper brain centers, the animal can be made to feel sleepy, thirsty, or hungry.

ESB by remote control has caused cats in Dr. Delgado's laboratory to eat ten times as much as they normally would. These "fat cats" will continue to gorge themselves as long as the hunger-controlling areas of their brains are stimulated. Stimulation of a nearby area, on the other hand, will turn off the hunger drive. Cats who are eating when this new area is stimulated will spit out their food in apparent disgust.

By stimulating other deep-rooted areas of the brain, an experimenter can control emotions such as fear, anger, and pleasure. A few years ago, Dr. Delgado demonstrated

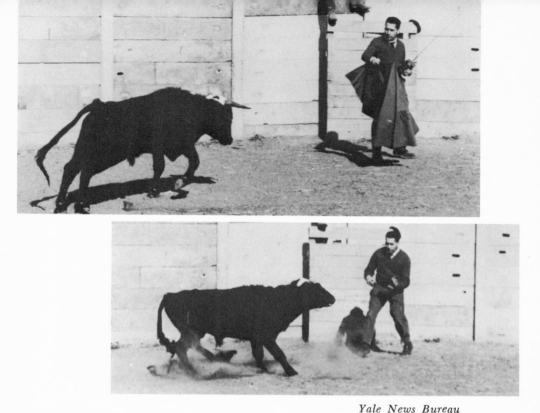

Dr. José Delgado and the fighting bull: the scientist pressed a button on a radio transmitter, and the bull screeched to a halt.

his behavior-control techniques by taking part in a "bull-fight" in Spain. Before the demonstration, electrodes were implanted in the brain of a powerful fighting bull who had been bred especially for fierceness. After the animal had recovered from this operation, Dr. Delgado climbed into the bull ring with him. Standing under a hot sun, the scientist waved a red cape. The bull glared at him, snorted and pawed the ground, lowered his head, and charged. Dr. Delgado waited as the bull bore down on him. Finally he pressed a small button on the radio transmitter in his hand. The bull screeched to a dusty halt. When the scientist pressed another button, the bull turned around and trotted peacefully away.

Social Revolution by Radio Waves

More recently, Dr. Delgado has used remote-control techniques to bring about changes in the social structure of a monkey colony. Like many other animals, rhesus monkeys are social creatures. Within a colony of these monkeys, each member has a certain social rank. His standing depends largely on how aggressive he is. The boss monkey wins his position as ruler by bullying his way to the top. With bared teeth, menacing growls, and other threatening motions he asserts his superiority over the rest of the colony. As its highest-ranking member, he reserves the best feeding and sleeping places for himself, has his pick of the females, and shows little patience with inferiors who get in his way.

Dr. Delgado selected a few typical monkey citizens on various levels of the social ladder. Electrodes implanted in their brains were connected to radio receivers strapped to their backs. Dr. Delgado soon demonstrated that he could change a monkey's social standing. By remote radio command, he could increase the aggressiveness of an inferior monkey and diminish the aggressiveness of a superior.

If the boss monkey's aggressiveness was turned off, the other monkeys were no longer afraid of him. The boss became so peaceable, in fact, his inferiors lost not only their fear but also their respect. They felt free to approach the boss and even get in his way. As soon as the radio signals stopped, however, the boss became as nasty as ever. Before long, the old dictator was in full control of the colony again.

During these experiments, Dr. Delgado found that inferior monkeys could learn to control the boss's aggressiveness just as scientists had done. A switch connected to a radio transmitter was set up just outside the monkey's cage. Within a few days, monkeys who were attacked frequently by the boss learned to pull the switch whenever they were threatened. They seemed quite excited by the discovery that they could magically alter the boss's mood. Soon they were having a delightful time pulling the switch whenever the boss glared at them.

"The old dream of an individual overpowering the strength of a dictator by remote control has come true," says Delgado. "At least, in our monkey colonies."

Similar experiments have been conducted at the Yerkes Regional Primate Research Center in Atlanta, Georgia. There, a timid male monkey, an aggressive male, and a female were placed together in a cage. The female quickly selected the more aggressive male as her partner. She even assisted him in taunting and threatening the inferior male. When this relationship was firmly established, scientists used radio signals to stimulate the aggressiveness of the inferior male. He immediately underwent a personality change. Instead of retreating to a corner of the cage, he began to stand his ground and fight back. After a while, he even started a few scuffles himself. As his radio-controlled aggressiveness persisted, the female changed her behavior too. At first, she withdrew to one side of the cage and simply watched. Finally she switched her allegiance. She sided with the once-timid male in attacks against her old partner, who had lost his standing as ruler of the cage.

The same experiment was repeated with many other monkeys placed in similar groups of two males and one female. In almost every case, the female proved to be fickle. She switched from one male to the other as their social standing changed.

Atlas of a Bird Brain

At the Max Planck Institute in Germany, scientists are compiling a three-dimensional atlas of a chicken's brain. When the atlas is finally completed, it will show in precise detail the location, size, and shape of the various brain centers that control chicken behavior.

Chickens were chosen for this project because they display such a rich inventory of instinctive behavior patterns. Much of their behavior can be predicted in advance since it consists of acts that are performed quite automatically, in a fixed manner. The "language" of chickens, for example, is made up of several dozen sounds, each having its own meaning. A chicken's ability to utter the right sound in the right situation is inborn and does not depend on learning or experience. Even chickens that are totally deaf from birth develop the complete vocabulary of "chickeneese."

Chickens maintain a rigid social order among themselves. It is known as the "pecking order" because it is actually based upon who gets to peck whom. Chickens of high social standing can peck their inferiors without fear of being pecked in return. This no-nonsense social ranking is established as the result of fights early in life, or when a flock is brought together for the first time.

High-ranking hens are entitled to be first when it comes time for feeding. They reserve for themselves the best roosting places in the hen house and are given the right-of-way when moving among the other chickens in the flock. Violators of this social code are punished by having their heads pecked or their feathers pulled by higher-ranking members of the flock.

It is always a rooster who rules the roost, if a rooster is present. Otherwise the honor goes to the highest-ranking hen. When there are several roosters in the chicken yard, they will fight among themselves for the highest position in barnyard society. Once the social order is established, and each chicken knows its place, the chicken yard remains a fairly stable and peaceful place.

Chickens at the Max Planck Institute behave just as chickens are supposed to behave, but not always of their own accord. Each chicken has a small plastic socket inserted permanently in its skull. Wire electrodes can be lowered through this socket down into any part of the chicken's brain. Since the brain is insensitive to touch, the electrodes cause no pain and can be put in place while

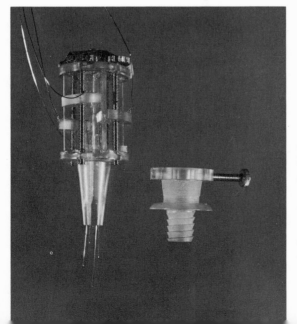

David Linton from
SCIENTIFIC AMERICAN

Stimulating apparatus: each chicken at the Max Planck Institute has a small plastic socket (right) inserted permanently in its skull. An electrode carrier (right) fits into the socket. The carrier holds four wire electrodes which can be lowered painlessly into various parts of the chicken's brain.

the chicken is fully conscious. Connected to the electrodes is a tiny radio receiver, weighing less than an ounce, which the chicken wears around its neck. And high above the chicken yard, radar-like antennas beam radio signals to individual chickens.

By stimulating different areas of a chicken's brain, experimenters at the Max Planck Institute can trigger almost any kind of typical chicken behavior. A chicken can be commanded to walk, jump, scratch, preen, ruffle its feathers, lift its wings, and so on. It can be made to cluck softly, to sound an alarm call, and to utter all the other sounds that make up a chicken's vocabulary. By remote radio control, a chicken can be directed to run over to a lower-ranking member of the flock and peck its head or pull its feathers. If no victim is available when the chicken receives this signal, it will look frantically about and will finally deliver a few excited pecks to the ground, like an angry child stamping his feet.

In some experiments, scientists have stimulated two different areas of the brain at once, triggering two different kinds of behavior. For example, a chicken may be directed to lift its wings as it pecks at the ground, or to preen its feathers as it turns around. If possible, the chicken will perform both acts at the same time. But what happens if the two acts conflict? Suppose the chicken is directed to turn to the right and to the left at the same time? In that case, nothing happens. Opposing urges will often cancel each other out. Sometimes, however, when a chicken is stimulated to perform two opposing acts at the same time, it will attempt to do so.

One hen was stimulated with the urge to attack; at the

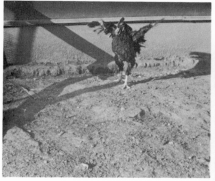

Lifting wings

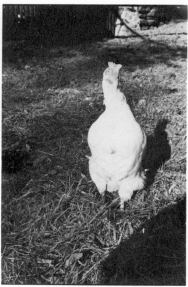

James E. Morriss
Chicken behavior:

stretching neck

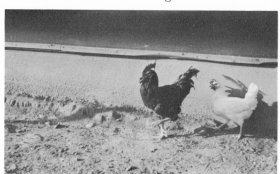

hen following rooster

same time she was stimulated with the urge to flee. She ruffled her feathers, spread her wings, let out a piercing cry, and began to run back and forth. If the hen had actually seen an enemy approaching her chicks, she might have behaved in the same way. Under these circumstances, the urge to attack and the urge to flee would both exist at the same time.

Some urges, or drives, are more powerful than others. Brain stimulation by remote control enables scientists to measure the strength of these drives by comparing them with each other. If two conflicting drives are stimulated at the same time, and one is stronger than the other, then the stronger drive will overcome the weaker one. After a while, however, the weaker drive may suddenly express itself.

This happened when a hen was stimulated both to sit down and to run away. At first, the urge to sit was more powerful, and that's what the hen did. But as the brain stimulation continued, the sitting hen seemed to become nervous, as if the urge to run was gradually building up. Suddenly, the hen jumped up from where she was sitting and fluttered away. Similar behavior might occur under natural conditions. If a hen who was sitting on her eggs

By stimulating different areas of a chicken's brain, experimenters can trigger almost any kind of behavior. Stimulation of one area of the brain causes a hen to flatten her feathers and stretch her neck (a). Stimulation of a different area causes the hen to fluff out her feathers (b). When both areas are stimulated at the same time, the stronger drive overcomes the weaker one; again, the hen flattens her feathers and stretches her neck. As soon as the stimulation ends, however, the weaker drive expresses itself and the hen suddenly fluffs her feathers (c). *From "Electrically Controlled Behavior," E. Von Holst and Ursula von Saint Paul. Copyright © 1962 by Scientific American, Inc. All rights reserved.*

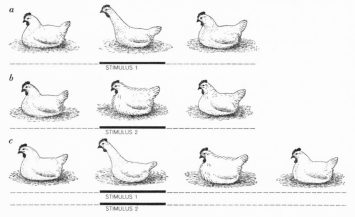

was threatened by danger, she would be reluctant to leave her nest until the last minute.

Can the brain tell the difference between nerve impulses that occur naturally and those that are triggered by a scientist's radio transmitter? A chicken being chased by a dog appears to be scared out of its wits. Yet the chicken seems just as frightened if a certain area of its brain is stimulated by remote control. Does this mean that the chicken actually "sees" an enemy? Can brain stimulation produce hallucinations? Some experiments indicate that it may.

Scientists at the Max Planck Institute implanted electrodes in the part of a chicken's brain that controls a specific kind of fear—the fear of ground enemies such as dogs and cats. As the chicken pecked for seeds, experimenters stimulated this area of the brain with a weak electric current. The chicken immediately stopped eating and stretched its neck, peering into the distance as if looking for danger. Gradually, the current was increased, and now the chicken grew nervous and excited as if it actually saw an enemy approaching. Just as the chicken began to flutter away in an effort to escape, the experimenters cut off the current, stopping the brain stimulation. The chicken seemed confused and perplexed. It peered about, as if looking for a dangerous creature that had suddenly disappeared.

In another experiment, electrodes were implanted in the same brain area, but this time two chickens were used. By means of a special amplifier, the scientists were able to establish radio contact between the brains of the two birds. Any electrical activity that occurred in one brain would be transmitted automatically to the brain of the other chicken.

The chickens were now placed in two separate rooms. Shortly afterwards, a dog on a leash was led into one of the rooms. The chicken in that room squawked in alarm, flapped its wings, and fluttered frantically up the wall.

Although no dog entered the second room, the chicken there behaved in the same way. As signals from the excited brain of the first chicken flashed messages of fear to the brain of the second chicken, who was alone in a quiet room, it too squawked in alarm, flapped its wings, and fluttered up the wall.

Benefits of Behavior Control

Janet was a charming and attractive twenty-year-old girl. She made friends easily and got along well with everyone—until she was overwhelmed by one of her terrible attacks. Then, for no apparent reason, she would fly into a violent and destructive tantrum. On more than a dozen occasions she had assaulted people with knives or scissors, and twice she had stabbed them seriously. After her attacks had subsided, she always felt confused, guilt-stricken, and deeply depressed.

She was suffering from a severe brain disorder which results in explosive seizures of uncontrollable rage. Since these seizures were both dangerous and unpredictable, Janet was finally committed to a hospital for the criminally insane. Had it not been for new techniques of ESB —electrical stimulation of the brain—she might have remained behind institutional walls for the rest of her life.

As it turned out, she became one of the first human patients to experience brain stimulation by remote control. Hoping to locate the source of her violent seizures, doctors implanted electrodes inside her brain and connected them to a small electronic device which was anchored to her skull. This device, called a *stimoceiver,* had been developed by Dr. José Delgado at Yale. Though it weighs less than an ounce and is no bigger than a button, it is both a brain stimulator and a brain-wave receiver. It can receive EEG recordings and can deliver electrical impulses to the brain by remote radio command.

As Janet moved freely about the hospital ward, doctors were able to study her brain-wave patterns and were also able to stimulate certain areas of her brain. Eventually they pinpointed the area that seemed responsible for her seizures. One afternoon, as the girl sat alone in her room, playing the guitar and singing softly to herself, doctors flashed a radio signal to the stimoceiver on her skull. Electrical impulses surged into the suspect area of her brain. Suddenly she flung her guitar across the room and in a fit of rage began to beat violently at the wall. The trouble-making cells in her brain had been identified. Soon afterwards, she underwent an operation in which those cells were destroyed, enabling her to lead a more normal life.

Today, people suffering from uncontrollable attacks of rage can often be treated successfully without surgery. Through ESB, doctors can not only identify the troubled area of the brain but can in some cases turn the patient's rage on and off at will. Epilepsy, severe depression, involuntary musclar spasms, and other serious mental and nervous disorders are also being treated by means of brain stimulation techniques. Of course, doctors are reluctant to implant electrodes deep within a human brain except in cases of urgent medical necessity. And yet many patients have worn electrodes for long periods of time, receiving systematic brain stimulation in the hospital or at outpatient clinics.

"The prospect of leaving wires inside the thinking brain might seem barbaric, uncomfortable, and dangerous," says Dr. Delgado, "but actually the patients who have undergone this experience have had no ill effects. In some cases, they have enjoyed a normal life as outpatients, returning to the clinic for periodic stimulations. Some of the women proved the adaptability of the feminine spirit to all situations by designing pretty hats to conceal their electronic headgear."

In fact, it is now possible for certain patients to control the symptoms of their illnesses by stimulating their own brains. This is accomplished by means of a transistor signaling device, the *intracranial self-stimulator* or ICSS. It can be carried on the belt or in a pocket or purse. Signals transmitted by the ICSS are picked up by an electronic socket on the patient's skull and are converted into electrical impulses. An epileptic patient, for example, can press a button on the stimulator when he feels a convulsive seizure coming on—sending stimulation to his brain and blocking the seizure before it starts. A patient with narcolepsy, or uncontrollable sleepiness, can press a button and stimulate himself into alert wakefulness. And a patient afflicted with bouts of suicidal depression can press a button and magically lift his mood.

Although devices such as the ICSS are still in the experimental stage, they are being used by several major

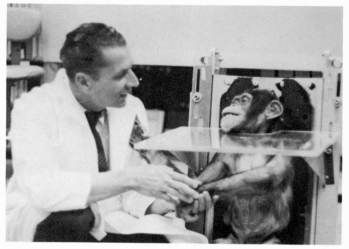

Dr. José Delgado and Paddy the chimp.

hospitals and have already benefited many patients. "Brain stimulation could lead to the relief of much human suffering, and to new treatments for mental and nervous disorders," says Dr. David Hamburg, chairman of the psychiatry department at Stanford University. "It could possibly help to solve some human problems, and it may ultimately affect man's understanding and conception of himself."

The Brain Tomorrow

Not long ago, newspapers around the world carried the story of an historic experiment conducted by Dr. José Delgado at Holloman Air Force Base in New Mexico. Dr. Delgado succeeded in establishing two-way radio contact between a computer and the brain of a chimpanzee named Paddy. The purpose of the experiment was to see if the natural aggressiveness of a young male chimp could be modified or perhaps eliminated by computer control.

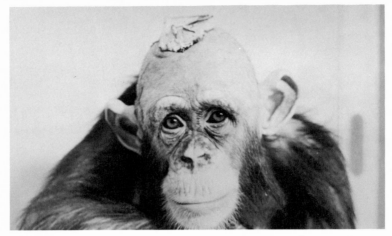

Yale News Bureau

Computer-brain hookup: a stimoceiver anchored to Paddy's skull broadcasts brain-wave recordings to a distant computer. The computer, in turn, radioes signals back to Paddy's brain, making him suppress his aggressive urges.

To begin with, 100 electrodes were implanted in Paddy's brain. A stimoceiver anchored to his skull broadcast brain-wave readings to the nearby computer. As the experiment proceeded, Paddy was allowed to roam freely on a small island in company with three other chimps. As he ran and played, ate and slept, the computer monitored his brain waves. It had been programmed to detect any brain-wave patterns that might indicate the beginnings of an aggressive mood.

Whenever Paddy felt aggressive, the computer radioed its own signals to an area of his brain that produced unpleasant and disturbing sensations when stimulated. In this way, the computer acted as an electronic conscience, punishing the chimp's brain as soon as aggressive urges appeared. Within two hours after the experiment began, brain-wave activity associated with aggressiveness dropped by fifty percent. Within a few days, these brain waves had almost entirely disappeared. Paddy's behavior had changed too. Instead of becoming involved in squabbles and fights with the other young chimps, he sat peacefully with his companions and responded calmly when visitors came to observe the experiment.

Dr. Delgado believes that in the near future similar computer-brain hookups may be used to treat human illnesses such as Parkinson's disease and epilepsy. Such a hookup might also be used to alleviate uncontrollable obsessions, fears, and anxieties, and to "nip in the bud" anti-social acts such as violent behavior.

Many mental and nervous disorders are characterized by unique brain-wave patterns. In epilepsy, for instance, slow, high-voltage brain waves warn of the gathering storm taking place in the brain. These waves begin to appear long before the onset of an epileptic fit. A patient's brain-wave activity could be monitored constantly by a distant computer, or even by a mini-computer carried on the body. The computer would recognize an impending attack and would respond by triggering radio stimulation to the affected area of the brain. A patient walking down the street might in this way avoid a convulsive seizure without even knowing it.

While the future medical benefits of ESB are highly promising, there are disturbing questions to be considered too. It is one thing to manipulate the brain of a suffering patient, enabling him to lead a more normal life. But it is something else again to manipulate the brain as a means of controlling human behavior. "It is not too early," warns Dr. Robert S. Morison of the Rockefeller Foundation, "to prepare ourselves for the day when there will be a behavioral science which will make possible the control of human behavior with a high degree of precision."

The power to control men's minds presents awesome

and far-reaching problems. Some scientists foresee the possibility of a nightmarish future when human infants might have hundreds of microelectrodes implanted permanently in their brains. The growing child's behavior would be monitored and controlled by a local switchboard or headquarters which would transmit instructions to all the human receivers in its area. Local headquarters would receive instructions from regional transmitters, which in turn would be directed by radio commands from a central headquarters. At each level, the transmitting stations would be operated by individuals whose privileged position in the society would allow them to have fewer and fewer electrodes implanted in their brains. Those in command of central headquarters would have no electrodes in their heads and would control the behavior of their fellow humans by virtue of their "superior wisdom."

It is little wonder that brain researchers tend to worry about the implications of their work. Dr. José Delgado has a more hopeful view of the future. Along with many other scientists, he argues that human behavior is much too complex to be controlled on any significant scale by remote radio command. On the contrary, advances in brain research may help us find intelligent solutions to difficult problems that have always confronted human beings. "Investigators will not be able to prevent the clash of conflicting desires or ideologies, but they can discover the mechanisms of anger, hate, and aggressiveness," says Dr. Delgado, "providing clues for the direction of more sociable and less cruel human beings."

If our growing mastery of the brain is to benefit man

rather than enslave him, it is important that ordinary citizens as well as scientists keep themselves informed about future advances in brain research. Yesterday's science fiction is fast becoming reality. How we deal with that reality today will shape our destiny tomorrow.

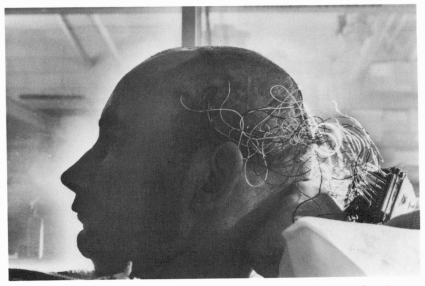

John Loengard, LIFE *Magazine* © *Time Inc.*

With 110 electrodes implanted in his head, this patient is undergoing electrical stimulation of the brain.

For Further Reading

BOOKS

Asimov, I., *The Human Brain*. New York, Signet Science Book Library, 1965. (Paperback)

Barnett, S. A., *Instinct and Intelligence*. Englewod Cliffs, N.J., Prentice-Hall, 1967.

Cosgrove, M., *The Strange World of Animal Senses*. New York, Dodd-Mead, 1961.

Delgado, J. M. R., *Physical Control of the Mind*. New York, Harper & Row, 1969.

Droscher, V., *The Mysterious Senses of Animals*. New York, E. P. Dutton, 1965.

Freedman, R. and Morriss, J. E., *Animal Instincts*. New York, Holiday House, 1970.

Freedman, R. and Morriss, J. E., *How Animals Learn*. New York, Holiday House, 1969.

Galambos, R., *Nerves and Muscles*. New York, Anchor Books, 1962. (Paperback)

Groch, J., *You and Your Brain*. New York, Harper & Row, 1963.

Hyde, M., *Your Brain: Master Computer*. New York, McGraw-Hill, 1964.

Nathan, P., *The Nervous System*. Philadelphia, J. P. Lippincott, 1969.

Pfeiffer, J., *The Human Brain*. New York, Pyramid Books, 1962. (Paperback)

Rosenfeld, A., *The Second Genesis*. Englewood Cliffs, N.J., Prentice-Hall, 1969.

Taylor, G., *The Biological Time Bomb*. New York, New American Library, 1968.

Vernon, J., *Inside the Black Room*. New York, Clarkson N. Potter, 1963.

Walter, W. G., *The Living Brain*. New York, W. W. Norton, 1963 (Paperback)

Wilson, J. R., *The Mind*. New York, Time-Life Books, 1969.

Wooldridge, D. E., *The Machinery of the Brain*. McGraw-Hill, 1963. (Paperback)

ARTICLES FROM *SCIENTIFIC AMERICAN*

Agranoff, B. W., "Memory and Protein Synthesis." June, 1967.

Atkinson, R. C., and Shiffrin, R. M., "The Control of Short-Term Memory." August, 1971.

Brazier, M. A. B., "The Analysis of Brain Waves." June, 1962.

French, J. D., "The Reticular Formation." May, 1957.

Gazzaniga, M., "The Split Brain in Man." August, 1967.

Gerard, R. W., "What Is Memory?" September, 1953.

Gray, G. W., "The Great Ravelled Knot." October, 1948.

Harlow, F. and Harlow, K., "Learning to Think." August, 1949.

Heron, W., "The Pathology of Boredom." January, 1957.

Holst, E. V. and Saint Paul, U. V., "Electrically Controlled Behavior." March, 1962.

Jouvet, M., "The States of Sleep." February, 1967.

Katz, B., "The Nerve Impulse." November, 1952.

Luria, A. R., "The Functional Organization of the Brain." March, 1970.

Muntz, W. R. A., "Vision in Frogs." March, 1964.

Olds, J., "Pleasure Centers in the Brain." October, 1956.

Peterson, L. R., "Short-Term Memory." July, 1966.

Pribram, K. H., "The Neurophysiology of Remembering." January, 1969.

Snider, R. S., "The Cerebellum." August, 1958.

Walter, W. G. "The Electrical Activity of the Brain." June, 1954.

Index